21 80
Z+HB
2794

Nan Ke

Male Urology and Sexual Dysfunction

中醫男科

A Handbook of TCM Urology & Male Sexual Dysfunction

by
Anna Lin

Blue Poppy Press

Published by:

BLUE POPPY PRESS
1775 LINDEN AVE.
BOULDER, CO 80304

FIRST EDITION
OCTOBER 1992

ISBN 0-936185-36-8
Library of Congress #92-073392

Printed at Westview Press, Boulder, CO on acid free, recycled paper with soy based ink

Published by Blue Poppy Press, Boulder, CO

Cover calligraphy by Zhang Ting-liang

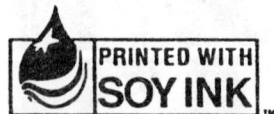

10 9 8 7 6 5 4 3 2

Editor's Preface

Nan ke is to men what *fu ke* or gynecology is to women. *Nan* means man or male. *Ke* means -ology, specialty, department, or the study of. In clinical practice, however, we can translate *nan ke* as male urology. The *nan ke* specialist diagnoses and treats diseases of the male urogenital organs. This includes urinary diseases and reproductive and sexual disorders.

In the People's Republic of China today, *nan ke* or male urology is a hot topic amongst TCM practitioners. In the last few years, *nan ke* hospitals, clinics, and research centers have been built and a number of *nan ke* books have been published. It is interesting that this recent Chinese interest in male urology parallels the emergence of the men's movement in the West.

To date, Blue Poppy Press has published a number of books on TCM *fu ke* or gynecology. However, little exists in the English language TCM literature on *nan ke* or male urology. When Anna Lin, an instructor at Samra University, asked if Blue Poppy Press would be interested in publishing a book on *nan ke*, I was immediately interested in her proposal. TCM does offer a number of effective, noniatrogenic, low cost treatments for the most common urogenital complaints and we are happy to be able to make these available to Western practitioners of TCM and their patients.

Ms. Lin has written this book based on a number of contemporary Chinese *nan ke* sources. It is meant as an introductory text to the clinical practice of TCM male urology. For years it has been our dream and intention to create such basic texts and clinical manuals for all the clinical specialties of TCM so that Western TCM education might attain true doctoral scope and status. With the publication of this book, one more such text exists on one more clinical specialty. Hopefully this book will serve as the basis for the incorporation of classes on male urology in Western acupuncture/Chinese medical schools. Until such schools offer classes in each of the clinical specialties of TCM, such as *nei ke*/internal medicine, *fu ke*/gynecology & obstetrics, *er ke*/pediatrics, *shang ke*/traumatology, *wai ke*/external medicine, *pi fu ke*/dermatology, *nan ke*/male urology, *zhong liu ke*/oncology, *yan ke*/opthalmology, *shen jing jing shen ke*/neurology/psychiatry, *kou qiang er bi hou ke*/ENT, and *lao nian ke*/geriatrics, our Western clinical education in TCM is far from professionally complete. This clinical manual should also help Western practitioners of TCM already in practice more knowledgably and confidantly treat male urogenital dysfunction.

Historically within Chinese medicine, specialization was primarily the province of the *ling yi* or itinerant, empirical practitioners and the *ru yi* or Confucian scholar-doctors tended to look down on such practice as a *xiao dao* or little *dao*. This meant a technical skill practiced for financial gain. It is also true that the basic conceptual framework of TCM as a specific style of Chinese medicine developed mostly out of this Confucian practice of medicine. However, although TCM diagnosis and treatment stresses taking into account the entire patient as the ground of their disease, nonetheless, there is the tendency in modern TCM to specialize. As long as the practitioner has a good conceptual grasp of the entirety of TCM theory and clinical practice, I believe such specialization is healthy since it allows for the relatively speedy development of penetrating insight and clinical efficacy in a limited group of diseases.

Rather than spreading oneself too thin and relying mostly on available textbooks and clinical manuals for textbook solutions, by specializing, one can gain special, concentrated experience and expertise in a more limited range of diseases. My teacher, Prof. Ding Ji-feng, once said that if one could treat even just frozen shoulder effectively most of the time, their rice bowl would never be empty. Personally, I have found this very good advice, and, as male baby boomers begin to age, *nan ke* or male urology is going to become a more and more important specialty within the Western practice of TCM.

As with our other recent Blue Poppy Press publications, we have used Wiseman and Boss' Chinese medical terminology as found in their *Glossary of Chinese Medical Terms and Acupuncture Points.* Medicinal identifications are given in Latin pharmacological nomenclature followed by pinyin in parentheses. We have chosen this method of identifying TCM medicinals both for its accuracy and unambiguity, its universality, and its credibility in the eyes of other medical professionals.

Some of the formulas listed in this book include dosages of individual ingredients. Others do not. This depends upon the Chinese source and whether doses were included in the source text. In any case, the dosages that are included are meant only for reference. Just as the formulas themselves are only meant as a guide and should not be prescribed necessarily as they appear in this book, so dosages must be decided upon individually, depending upon the signs and symptoms of each patient. Unless one already has a command of the *materia medica* and is proficient at analyzing and writing prescriptions, one should be careful using the formulas which appear in this text by rote. If one is not clear about the appropriate amounts of ingredients in those formulas for which no amounts are given, even more care should be taken when attempting to use this book.

Acupuncture points are identified first by their Chinese name rendered in pinyin followed by their numerical notation. For regular channel points we have used the numbering system found in *Essentials of Chinese Acupuncture & Moxibustion*. For non-channel points, we have used the numbering system found in *Acupuncture: A Comprehensive Text*. This book is divided into two sections. The first presents the basic theory of TCM *nan ke* and the second covers the diagnosis and treatment of the most common *nan ke* complaints.

Bob Flaws
Boulder, CO
April 7, 1992

Contents

Book Two
The Treatment of Urological & Male Sexual Dysfunction Diseases

Book One

The Theory of TCM Urology & Male Sexual Dysfunction

The Causes of Sexual Dysfunction

According to Traditional Chinese Medicine, disease may be caused by internal, external, or neither internal nor external causes. Internal causes specifically refer to the seven passions. External causes specifically refer to the six evils. While neither internal nor external causes may refer to lifestyle and dietary improprieties but also include traumatic injury. In addition, disease, including sexual dysfunction may also be caused by congenital insufficiency.

The seven passions

The seven passions include joy, anger, worry, melancholy, grief, fear, and fright. These reflect one's internal response to the external stimuli provoked by their interaction with the world. When these become extreme or are inappropriate or prolonged, they affect the various internal organs adversely and thus cause disease. Excessive anger, for example, can injure the liver. Excessive joy injures the heart. Excessive worry and brooding injure the spleen. Excessive melancholy and grief injure the lungs. Excessive fear injures the kidneys.

Because anger leads to counterflow ascent of the qi, emotional overtaxation due to anger causes disturbance in the flow of liver qi. This may then manifest as chest fullness, redness of the eyes, rapid breathing, a greenish white facial color, and even hematemesis and fainting. Because anger injures its corresponding organ, the liver, its qi fails to disperse. This, in turn, may result in menstrual disorders in women and spermatorrhea in men. Additionally, it may also result in impotence and premature ejaculation. Excessive anger and/or depression also result in mental dysfunction which may thence obstruct or retard sexual function causing a reduction in sexual drive or libido.

Worry can cause qi stagnation which may then manifest as a decline in appetite, insomnia, or manic depressive types of behavior. Untreated disorders of this type can cause retardation or obstruction of sexual function, resulting in decrease of libido or sexual drive.

When people are under severe emotional stress, it is not uncommon for them to suffer from impotence and a decrease in libido. Sadness and sorrow can injure the lungs and dissipate or scatter the qi, with symptoms of a pale or lusterless face, fatigue, sighing, crying, and decreased sexual drive.

Fear causes the qi to descend. This may damage the kidney qi resulting in urinary incontinence, impotence, spermatorrhea, etc., whereas fright causes the qi to be chaotic and frightful. Shocking conditions disturb the *shen* or spirit. This results in all kinds of sexual dysfunction or obstruction/retardation.

Joy, on the other hand, renders the qi flow sluggish, and patients may suffer from shortness of breath with various sexual difficulties.

Further, stagnancy and depression of the qi may transform into fire — liver fire, heart fire, lung fire, stomach fire, or kidney fire. These fires can damage and injure the body fluids and damage kidney *jing* or essence. Injury of kidney *jing* results in kidney yin vacuity and may manifest in sexual dysfunction.

Lifestyle

In TCM, harmful lifestyle includes improper lifestyle, stress, and improper diet.

It is said in the *Su Wen*, "Excessive lying injures the qi; sitting too long injures the flesh; staring too long (as in reading) injures the blood; standing too long injures the bones; and walking too long injures the sinews." This line suggests that either overwork or underwork may cause imbalances in the qi and blood, sinews and bones, muscles and flesh, and, by extension, in the organs and bowels. Since the sexual organs are connected to the organs and bowels and are irrigated and nourished by the qi, blood, and body fluids, lifestyle improprieties may thus result in sexual dysfunction as well as other types of disease.

Improper diet includes both over- and underconsumption. For instance, overeating fatty, oily foods or drinking too much may result in food stagnation and its further transformation into heat, dampness, or phlegm, thus causing various disorders which may eventually affect sexual function. Overconsumption of spicy foods or yang-supplementing foods can stir up and arouse the yang, causing injury to the *jing* essence and disrupting sexual function. Overeating and overdrinking injure the spleen and stomach in turn bringing about qi and blood vacuity. This then causes an insufficiency of *jing* essence and thus, characteristically, sexual dysfunction or decreased sexual function. Likewise, not eating enough may also injure the spleen and stomach with the same consequences. Overconsumption of cold, raw foods, including habitually drinking cold liquids, may injure yang. Vacuity of kidney yang results in a reduction of *ming men* fire and thence a decline in sexual function and desire.

Therefore, having a balanced and proper lifestyle and diet are the keys to maintaining a healthy body and, as an extension of this, healthy sexual desire and function.

The six evils

Wind, cold, summer heat, dampness, dryness, and fire are called the six qi when they are normal. As such, they represent the normal changes in weather and season of the macrocosmic world.

However, when these six qi are either inappropriate or excessive, they are then called the six evils and may cause disease, including harm to one's sexual function.

Wind is believed the leader of all these external pathogens or evils. It is said that wind is the beginning of a hundred diseases. Typically, wind-related disorders are further complicated by accompanying dampness, cold, or heat. Wind diseases are characterized by sudden onset and constant migration and change. The clinical manifestations of wind- related disorders pertaining to sexual function include itching of the external genitalia and pain and/or swelling caused by wind heat. Wind as an external pathogen or evil is considered a yang factor.

Evil cold is usually characterized as a yin factor. It impairs and impedes the yang qi of the body, thus obstructing the flow of qi and blood. This causes such urogenital diseases as scrotal spasm and pain in combination with other, systemic cold pattern symptoms such as aversion to cold, cold limbs, abdominal pain, profuse, clear urine, and low back pain.

Evil heat or fire is a yang factor which injures the yin fluids of the body. It may also result in reckless movement of *jing* or blood. Examples of heat-related urogenital injury include sterility or sexual dysfunction brought about by increased temperature of the scrotum or testes, for instance by soaking for too long in a hot bath.

Dampness is a heavy, turbid, sticky, lingering evil. It is a yin factor which usually affects the lower body and especially the sexual organs. It often causes itching of the genitalia. Dampness also has a tendency to recur.

Dryness as an external evil or pathogen mostly appears in the dry autumn season. It may manifest as dry skin, dry nose, dry lips, dry throat, dry cough, dry stools, etc. Dryness injures yin and body fluids. It may also give rise to vacuity heat. Dry heat accumulating in or injuring the lungs may cause problems with the lungs descension of body fluids and/or their nourishing of the kidneys and thence to the control and consolidation of urine and *jing*.

Amongst the six evils, those most typically responsible for causing disease and especially diseases of the urogenital organs and sexual dysfunction are cold, dampness, and heat.

Traumatic injury

Traumatic injury may directly injure the genitalia or indirectly injure the *chong, ren, du*, or *dai* vessels. Such injury may cause disharmony between the *jing* and blood and thus sexual dysfunction.

Congenital insufficiency

Congenital insufficiency may cause sexual dysfunction as well as result in various congenital abnormalities of the reproductive organs and tract. In men, these are classically referred to as the *wu bu nan* or the "five not men" and in women the *wu bu nu*, the "five not women". These are five congenital abnormalities of the reproductive organs in men and women respectively which render them either infertile or incapable of normal sexual relations. In men these include *tian* or congenital lack of testes, *lou* or habitual emission, *jian*, malformation of the genitalia or castration, *qie*, impotence, and *bian* or hermaphrodism.

正氣存內，邪不
可干。
"素問·刺法論"

If righteous qi is kept inside,
evil qi cannot invade.

The Disease Mechanisms of Sexual Dysfunction

Kidney disorders

In TCM, functional disorders of the kidneys may relate to a variety of disorders, such as urinary problems, genital disorders, internal secretory disorders, and central nervous system disorders. The kidneys are referred to as the organ of fire and water. This means that they contain both *yuan yang* or original yang, *i.e.*, kidney yang, and *yuan yin*, original or kidney yin. The kidneys' major function according to TCM is storing the *jing* essence. Birth, growth, maturation, and decline and death all have a close relationship to kidney qi and *jing* and this includes sexual maturation and sexual reproduction in particular.

The kidneys store two kinds of *jing* essence. One is the congenital or prenatal jing, the *xian tian zhi jing*. The other is the postnatal or acquired *jing*, the *hou tian zhi jing*. The congenital *jing* is also known as the reproductive *jing*, the *sheng zhi zhi jing*, while the postnatal *jing* is sometimes called *shui gu zhi jing*, the essence of water and grains. Another name for postnatal *jing* is the *zang fu zhi jing* or essence of the organs and bowels. Although these two types of *jing* essence each have their own source of generation and individual functions, there is also a reciprocal relationship between these two. Congenital essence is dependent upon the nutritional supplementation of the acquired essence. In turn, it is the *jing qi* which catalyzes the transformation of water and grains and thus it is said that the prenatal *jing* is the foundation of the postnatal *jing*.

Any imbalance in the kidneys' function of storing the *jing* may result in kidney qi vacuity, kidney yin vacuity, both kidney yin and yang vacuity, kidney spleen dual vacuity, or loss of communication between the kidneys and heart. And any of these may result in sexual dysfunction.

The kidneys also control the two yin and the opening and closing of the yin gates. The two yin refer to the vaginal/urethral meatus and anus in women and the urethral meatus and anus in men. In the case of men, the urethral opening is the front yin or *qian yin* and the anus is the back yin or *hou yin*, and it is the consolidating, securing function of the kidney qi which controls the opening and closing of these two yin gates. Thus, in this way as well, the kidneys have a direct control and relationship to urogenital function.

When kidney qi is vacuous, this leads to kidney yin or kidney yang vacuity and thence may result in sexual dysfunction or diseases of the urogenital region. The kidneys are also the root of the *chong* and *ren*. These two vessels are the two main vessels amongst the eight extraordinary vessels. All these vessels are controlled by the kidneys. Therefore it is said, "The *chong* is the sea of blood and the *ren* controls conception (or sexual reproduction)."

Further, the low back or lumbar region is the outer mansion of the kidneys. Flexibility in movement of the lumbar region depends upon sufficiency of kidney qi, whereas, exhaustion of kidney *jing* due to overwork or excessive sexual activity results in lumbar pain, soreness, and weakness.

The connection between the kidneys and the brain is evidenced by the kidneys' production of the bone and marrow. It is said in the *Su Wen*, "All bone marrow belongs to the brain." In addition, the brain is sometimes referred to as the sea of marrow, the *sui hai*. The brain is an extraordinary organ in the body. It is the supreme controller of mental functioning and activities. It controls and guides the various biological systems of the body. Through its control of the body's systems, it also has a profound effect on sexual function. According to Chinese medical theory, the marrow of the brain is dependent upon the *jing* essence of the kidneys.

In TCM, sufficiency of kidney *jing* and qi are necessary for proper brain function and for healthy mental activity conducive to a healthy sexual life. Kidney vacuity, whether of the qi or *jing*, leads to a condition of vacuity of the marrow. This results in lack of nutrients to the brain and that, in turn, may have an adverse effect on one's sexual function.

The fact the kidneys are intimately connected with sexual function and that their disease is intimately connected with sexual dysfunction is further supported and clarified by examining the empirical results of kidney supplementation on sexual function. TCM clinical experience and research suggest that there are five major functions of supplementing the kidneys.

1. Kidney supplementation helps prevent disease.

The body's absorption of qi is governed by the kidneys. Thus it is said that the kidneys are the root of all qi. *Yuan qi*, chest qi, *ying qi, wei qi,* and *zheng qi* are all governed by the kidneys. *Zheng qi* refers to the immune system of the body. The strength of the *zheng* or righteous qi helps the body counter the attack of external evils. However, if it is weak, this allows easy penetration by those same external evils. Thus it is said in the *Nei Jing*, "When *zheng qi* resides within the body, external evils can never attack." As seen above, attack by the six external evils can cause male urogenital diseases. Therefore, supplementing the kidneys can help prevent such disease. Supplementing the kidneys means to supplement the yin, yang, or qi of the kidneys.

2. Kidney supplementation enhances sexual function.

The kidneys store the *jing*, and the two types of *jing* mentioned above are closely connected. Congenital *jing* is specifically associated with the reproductive organs, such as the ovaries, scrotal contents, and other sexual glands, while the acquired *jing* relates to the essence of the organs and bowels, the *zang fu zhi jing*. Thus kidney supplementation can help improve bodily secretions, *i.e.*, hormonal secretions associated with sexual desire and function. For instance, such kidney supplements as Placenta Hominis (*Zi He Che*), Radix Morindae Officinalis (*Ba Ji Tian*), Radix Polygoni Multiflori (*He Shou Wu*), and Radix Praeparatus Aconiti Carmichaeli (*Fu Zi*) can adjust the adrenal or corticosteroid hormones, whereas kidney supplementing medicinals such as Cornu Cervi Parvum (*Lu Rong*), Semen Cnidii Monnieri (*She Chuan Zi*), and Herba Epimedii (*Yin Yang Huo*) have a similar effect on the sexual hormones. Further, it has been demonstrated clinically that supplementing kidney yin and warming kidney yang are effective for treating sex-related dysfunctions.

3. Kidney supplementation strengthens the body.

It is said that, "The kidneys hold the office of labor from whence agility emanates." Supplementing the kidneys helps fill kidney *jing* and boosts kidney qi, thus strengthening the entire body. It has been proven in China experimentally that kidney supplementation can help improve the metabolic function of the body, hence strengthening it. Those who are weak and exhausted tend not to have any energy to spare for sexual activity and reproduction. Bare survival biologically tends to take precedence over such endeavors. Therefore, a strong body helps ensure robust and normal sexual drive and function and supplementing the kidneys helps strengthen the body.

4. Kidney supplementation leads to longevity.

Chinese medicine has long believed that longevity is related to the strength and supply of *jing* essence and *yuan qi* stored in the kidneys. The majority of Chinese medicinals and formulas for promoting longevity are all kidney supplements. The first chapter of the *Su Wen* clearly relates length of life with kidney *jing*. On the other hand, these same medicinals and formulas are also used to promote sexual drive and function in the elderly. For instance, not only is Radix Polygoni Multiflori (*He Shou Wu*) credited with keeping Mr. He's hair black and prolonging his life, but is also credited with his siring of numerous offspring at an advanced age.

5. Kidney supplementation helps combat disease.

It is said in the *Nei Jing*, "When yin and yang are in equilibrium, the essence-spirit is balanced." Any imbalance in the equilibrium of the yin and yang results in a state of unhealthiness. TCM regards the root of all disorders as stemming from imbalance between yin and yang. Because the kidneys are the root of yin and yang in the body, supplementing the kidneys, whether yin or yang depending upon the circumstance, can help restore the equilibrium between yin and yang to the body and thus aid in the course of treating disease. On the one hand, kidney supplementation can help treat, specifically, diseases of the urogenital tract. On the other, by treating disease, *yuan qi* and *jing* essence are conserved, since long term illness depletes these two. Thus, by adjusting the balance of yin and yang through supplementing the kidneys and treating disease, sufficiency of these two can be maintained and aided and hence sexual drive and function.

The effects of kidney supplementation as described above are often seen in the course of treating sexual dysfunction and disability. Since male sexual dysfunction can result from the aging process, weakening of the body, and other related diseases, supplementing the kidneys helps improve immunity and prevents premature aging while at the same time helps to strengthen the sexual function.

Liver imbalance

The liver channel travels through the external genitalia and thus the liver has strong ties with the reproductive organs and many of their diseases. It is said, "The liver governs free coursing." In terms of its maintaining patency and free flow through the genitalia, it adjusts the forming of the sperm and body fluids. When healthy, the liver stores the blood and is associated with the formation of *jing* in men and blood in women. When diseased, imbalances in liver function typically result in liver qi stagnation. Stagnant liver qi may thence transform into fire. This fire may lead to insufficiency of liver blood, resulting in ascension of liver yang. Thus, sexual dysfunction may result from a number of liver disorders, including liver wind, damp heat in the liver channel, and ascension of liver yang.

Spleen vacuity

The spleen governs the qi of the middle burner. It is the source of generation and transformation. It produces and transforms the qi and blood. Surpluses of qi and blood are transformed into acquired essence which nourish the prenatal or reproductive essence. Thus diseases involving spleen vacuity can result eventually in essence insufficiency. Spleen qi also restrains the blood and *jing* essence. If spleen qi becomes insufficient, blood and/or *jing* may be lost involuntarily, while impairment of the spleen's functions of transportation and transformation may result in the generation of dampness and phlegm. This, being innately heavy and turbid, tends to percolate downward and may result in obstruction of the *jing shi* or palace of essence by water, phlegm, and/or damp turbidity. This may cause infertility and ejaculatory problems such as failure to ejaculate.

Heart vacuity

The heart's function is to govern the blood, control the *shen ming* or spiritual brilliance housing the spirit, and to control the mental activity including the sexual function and energy. It is said that only if the heart function is healthy can the rest of the body be balanced. Insufficiency of heart blood may lead to upward flaming of the heart fire. This may lead to a breakdown or rupture of communication between the heart and kidneys or dual vacuity of the heart and spleen qi. Either of these may result in sexual dysfunction.

Injury of the *chong, ren, du,* & *dai mai*

Each of these vessels has its own specific functions. The *chong mai* is the sea of blood. The *ren mai* controls conception and pregnancy. The *du mai* is the sea of yang and governs the *yuan qi* of the body. The *dai mai* is the belt which connects as well as constricts/restricts or controls all the other channels of the body, thus facilitating the smooth flow of qi and blood throughout the body. All four of these vessels are closely connected with the body's sexual function. They are also easily injured by the six evils, seven passions, and various disorders of the organs and bowels. Any direct or indirect injury of any of these four vessels may result in sexual dysfunction and disorders.

Qi & blood imbalances

Qi is the commander of the blood, while blood is the mother of qi. Qi and blood are thus mutually interdependent. Blood generates the *jing* essence and *jing* transforms into qi. Qi and blood circulate throughout the body supplying all its organs and bowels and its various tissues with nutrients. Imbalances resulting from qi and blood vacuity, qi stagnation and blood stasis, counterflow of qi, blood heat or cold blood may thus all result in sexual dysfunction or disease.

The Treatment of Sexual Dysfunction Based on the Discrimination of Patterns

Basing the treatment of disease on the discrimination of patterns is the foundation of the TCM methodology. This is called in Chinese *bian zheng lun zhi*. Using such a discriminaton of patterns as the guiding principle of treatment is no less so for the treatment of sexual and urological diseases as for any other. When attempting to discriminate patterns in the treatment of urogenital diseases one must take into account:

1. The location of the disease. This includes the concepts of *biao* or outside and *li* or inside, above and below.

2. The nature of the disease. This means whether the disease is characterized as replete or *shi* or vacuous or *xu,* and whether it is hot or cold.

3. The cause of the disease. Male urogenital diseases may be due in general to imbalances between yin and yang or be due to the struggle between evil and righteous qi. In particular, they may be due to the six evils, the seven passions, diet, lifestyle, or traumatic injury.

Arriving at a correct pattern discrimination diagnosis is crucial in the treatment of male urogenital diseases. Since, in TCM, treatment is primarily predicated upon the pattern discrimination diagnosis, a wrong pattern discrimination will lead to a categorically incorrect treatment plan. For instance, *Nan Bao* is a popular Chinese patent medicine. Its name means male treasure. It is indicated for spermatorrhea only if the underlying pattern of disharmony or cause is insufficiency of the kidneys' consolidating the *jing* essence. If, however, an individual's spermatorrhea is a direct result of liver gallbladder damp heat, this formula will not treat this patient's spermatorrhea, and may actually worsen their condition. In this case, the appropriate formula is *Long Dan Xie Gan Tang*. Another example is in the treatment of decreased sexual drive. *Shen Qi Wan* is another popular Chinese patent medicine. It treats decreased sexual drive, but only if that is caused by an underlying kidney yang vacuity. If caused by kidney yin vacuity, *Shen Qi Wan* will make the situation worse.

Thus it can be seen that the proper selection of medicinals in TCM for the treatment of urogenital disorders is predicated upon a correct *bian zheng* diagnosis. Based on such a diagnosis, one then logically states the treatment principles which will correct the imbalance implied in the name of the pattern. Then based on these principles, one chooses the correct formulas and medicinals. For instance, if a decrease in sexual drive is due to kidney yang vacuity, the therapeutic principles for rectifying that vacuity are to supplement the kidneys and to warm or strengthen yang. With those as one's guiding principles, one must pick a supplementing formula which specifically supplements the kidneys and warms yang. Any other formula or medicinals are categorically wrong in this case. At best, they will not help the patient and, at worst, they may make the patient sicker.

4

The Physical Characteristics of Aging in Men

The process of aging and its physical signs in men are different than in women. The aging process and the male climacteric occurs at a later age for men. Based on a passage from the *Nei Jing*, women's growth, maturation, decline and climacteric are measured in multiples of 7 years, whereas men's are measured in multiples of 8. According to Traditional Chinese Medicine, the aging process is the result of a decrease in the functional activities of the kidneys. The kidneys store the *jing* and are the root of the *yuan qi*. Repletion or vacuity of the kidneys is reflected in the quantity and quality of the *jing qi*. *Jing qi*'s function is to govern sexual function, the bones and marrow, the hair (on the head), and the strength of the teeth. Because the aging process results in the debility and decline of these very functions and tissues, thus it is said in Chinese medicine that insufficiency of *jing qi* results in the aging process. As a man turns 40 years old, the decline of kidney qi begins. Loose teeth, thinning hair, hair loss, and decreased sex drive are a few of the symptoms indicating kidney qi vacuity and decline.

Men are yang in nature. This yang nature is responsible for men's faster metabolic rate, stronger *zang fu* function, and increased mobility, all of which can lead to early exhaustion of *yuan qi* and weakness of kidney *jing qi*. *Jing* is the root of life and the source of the human body, and its condition greatly determines the extent of a person's life. In consuming the *jing*, a man consumes his life. Middle-aged and elderly men need to conserve their *jing* and avoid that which would lead to the loss of *jing*, most notably sex with ejaculation. Further, as *jing qi* becomes weaker due to age, various disease processes may also commence, since *jing* is the root of yin and yang and the foundation of the body's metabolism.

The therapeutic principles for treating vacuity weaknesses of the *jing qi* include boosting kidney *jing*, consolidating the kidneys, replenishing the *jing* essence, supplementing the kidneys, strengthening kidney yang, and moistening kidney yin.

5

Heat Penetrating the Blood Chamber, the *Chong, Ren, & Du,* and Its Effect on Male Urology

In the minds of many, the *chong, ren,* and *du* are primarily related to problems of the female urogenital system. However, these vessels also play an important role in male sexual function and dysfunction. Traditional Chinese Medicine regards the scrotum and its contents as the palace of *jing.* Its contents store the sperm and control reproduction. According to the *Nei Jing,* by the time a man reaches his 16th birthday, the kidneys are flourishing, the *ren mai* is free and unobstructed (*tong*), and the *tai chong* or great penetrating vessel is full. This sets the stage for the production of sperm within the testes. The scrotum and testes are, therefore, closely related to the *chong, ren,* and *du mai.* In males, the *chong* and *ren* originate from the palace of *jing* or the scrotum/testes. According to TCM theory, the thoroughfares of the *chong, ren,* and *du* vessels are branches emanating from the palace of *jing.* Therefore, it is not unusual to treat male sexual dysfunction via treating these three vessels.

Likewise, heat entering the blood chamber has long been considered a female problem. In actual fact, men also suffer from this disorder. In men, the blood chamber is believed to be the liver, due to that organ's function of storing the blood and the *hun.* Heat entering and invading the blood chamber injures and damages the blood and yin. These in turn then fail to contain and restrain yang. The appropriate formula for treating this condition is *Xiao Chai Hu Tang* (Minor Bupleurum Decoction).

人與天地相參也，
與日月相應也。

「靈樞・歲露

Humans exist within heaven and earth
and therefore resonate with the sun and moon.

6

Conserving Men's Life

For men, conserving life essentially means conserving the *jing* essence, since *jing* is the material basis of life and it directly influences the growth and aging processes. A strong, healthy supply of *jing* assures a strong, healthy life and hence the aging process is retarded. A deficiency of *jing* leads to weakness of the life force. Therefore, to conserve and prolong their lives, men need to conserve their *jing* essence. TCM posits a number of ways a man can conserve and preserve his *jing* essence.

1. Controlling one's sexual drive

Controlling one's sexual drive does not mean total abstinence from sex. Rather it implies control and pacing of one's loss of reproductive essence during sex. Since the sperm is the physical manifestation of this reproductive essence, control and pacing means limiting the frequency of ejaculation. Even from a Western medical point of view, excessive ejaculation can lead to exhaustion of the testes with decrease in testicular size and a loss of zinc in the body. This then weakens the life force and speeds up the aging process.

Traditionally, there are a number of formulas or recipes for pacing one's ejaculation and conserving one's *jing*. According to Sun Si-miao, by the time one is in their 30s, they should ejaculate only once every couple of days. In their 40s, only once per week. In their 50s, only once every couple of weeks. Around 60, only once per month. And after 60, not at all. This regimen must also be tempered by season of the year (fall & winter less; spring &

summer more), constitution, and present condition. For instance, someone who is constitutionally weak and deficient should ejaculate less frequently, as should someone recuperating from disease. In addition, one should not ejaculate when excessively fatigued.

Because all schools and styles of Oriental medicine relate the ejaculate to the *jing* essence, and the *jing* essence to the maintenance of health and the slowing of the aging process, all schools and styles of Oriental medicine place great importance on regulating the male's ejaculatory frequency. This is why the Chinese medical literature addresses again and again such symptoms as spermatorrhea, nocturnal emissions, and premature ejaculation. This is an area which modern Western medicine does not address adequately but which is, nonetheless, an important area in terms of preserving one's health and lengthening one's life.

2. Calming the heart spirit

Within the human organism, the heart is the emperor or ruler. When the heart is calm and healthy, the organs and bowels of the entire body also tend to be healthy and strong. This then creates abundant *zang fu zhi jing*. In addition, when the heart is calm, sexual drive tends to be less. Conversely, when the heart spirit is agitated, this tends to disturb and inflame the *ming men*. This is based on the relationship between imperial and ministerial fire. Stirring of the *ming men zhi huo* in turn leads to increased sexual drive and a tendency to lose one's *jing* essence through ejaculation and spermatorrhea. Thus a calm heart spirit leads to the palace of *jing* being full and sufficient.

3. Avoiding masturbation

Based on the above TCM theory regarding the *jing* essence and the aging process, it is easy to see that loss of reproductive essence through masturbation is deleterious to one's health. In fact, excessive masturbation during one's youth can lead to premature weakening of one's kidneys which then manifests as disease or sexual dysfunction in one's late 30s and 40s. Therefore, men should avoid masturbating at no matter what age but especially as they get older.

4. Harmonizing the seven passions

Any of the seven passions, when extreme, can transform into fire. Fire injures the blood and yin, and the blood and yin are related to the *jing*. Thus emotional extremes can lead to damage and injury of the *jing* essence. In particular, anger most easily transforms into evil heat. This evil heat can not only waste the blood but also cause a failure in the liver's storing of the blood. This then may result in various hemorrhagic disorders. Because the blood and *jing* share a common source, this can also injure and exhaust the *jing*.

5. Maintaining a balance between labor and rest

Sufficient exercise improves the function of the spleen and stomach. Because the spleen and stomach are the postnatal root of qi and blood production, sufficient exercise leads to a catalyzation of qi and blood production. If qi and blood are abundant, their excess is transformed into acquired *jing* which is then stored in and bolsters the prenatal essence in the kidneys. Insufficient exercise, on the other hand, leads to a retardation of the flow of qi and blood, the tendency for phlegm and dampness to accumulate, and weakened spleen and stomach function. In this case, qi and blood are less abundant and *jing* production is not as great. Overexercise exhausts the qi and blood and consumes *jing* essence. Therefore, it is important to regulate and balance one's work and rest so as to maximize qi and blood production while minimizing its consumption. Thus the *jing* can remain healthy and full.

6. Preventing disease

Disease, especially if chronic or prolonged, tends to injure the *jing*. Therefore, preventing the arisal of disease is another method for conserving and preserving one's *jing* essence in healthy amounts. If one does become sick, one should seek early and comprehensive treatment so that the disease is not allowed to drag on, thus either impairing the production of postnatal or acquired *jing*, or consuming *jing qi*.

7. Supplementing with Chinese herbal medicinals

Kidney *jing* deficiency and weakness, whether congenital or acquired, can be supplemented by using the appropriate supplementing and nourishing medicinals. This is one of the great insights of Chinese medicine. As one ages, one should take appropriate supplementing medicinals in order to maintain a healthy spleen and stomach and nourish and strengthen kidney yin and yang. Thus both acquired and prenatal essences can be fulfilled and their sufficiency maintained. In particular, one should make use of supplementing medicinals in the winter.

8. Avoiding addictions & partialities

Smoking, drinking alcohol, and excessive consumption of greasy, spicy foods can all injure kidney *jing*. Smoking injures yin fluids and causes internal heat. This then wastes yin fluids and blood and injures the lungs. Because the lungs send down the qi to nourish the kidneys, poor lung function can directly weaken the kidneys. Because fluids and blood share a common source as do blood and *jing*, injury of lung fluids can waste and exhaust kidney yin and *jing* over time. Alcohol also tends to generate internal heat which likewise injures kidney yin and *jing*. In addition, alcohol weakens the spleen and generates dampness, thus obstructing the root of postnatal qi and blood and, therefore, acquired *jing* production. Greasy, spicy foods essentially do the same things.

In addition, one should maintain proper genital hygiene. Tight underwear should be avoided as this can increase one's sexual drive and lead to a consequent loss of reproductive essence. When ministerial fire becomes inflamed, *jing* essence is injured and damaged.

Further, one should also not eat too many bitter, cold or raw, chilly foods. These can douse the fire of digestion and harm the spleen and stomach's generation and transformation of qi and blood. Therefore, as one ages, it is best to eat clear, light or bland foods in small amounts frequently throughout the day so as to maximize the spleen and stomach's creation of qi and blood and thus acquired essence.

氣血心和，百病乃
變化而生。

「素問 · 調經論」

If qi and blood are not harmonious,
hundreds of disease changes and transformations may arise.

7

Treatment Methods & Formula Discussions

Zhi fa
Treatment methods

In TCM, the choice of treatment methods applied in urological disorders depends upon a discrimination of patterns rather than upon the patient's disease diagnosis. Choice of treatment principles (*zhi yuan*) or treatment methods (*zhi fa*) are the intermediate step between a pattern discriminaton diagnosis and selecting formulas and medicinals to rectify or remedy that pattern diagnosis. For instance, if the kidneys are found to be vacuous and deficient, the principle for their treatment is to supplement the kidneys. In that case, this principle leads one to select a formula from the supplementing category which specifically supplements the kidneys. Thus there is a logical and orderly progression from pattern diagnosis to statement of treatment principles or methods and thence to the selection and erection of a treatment plan. This three step methodology is the hallmark of TCM as a rational style of Chinese medicine.

1. Supplementing the kidneys

Urological and reproductive diseases are strongly related to the kidneys. The following treatment methods are applicable to kidney vacuity related problems.

A. Replenishing kidney *jing*

Kidney *jing* insufficiency may cause impotence and failure to ejaculate. The basic formula to treat this is *Zuo Gui Yin*.

Zuo Gui Yin

Fructus Lycii Chinensis (*Gou Qi Zi*)
Radix Coquitus Rehmanniae (*Shu Di*)
Fructus Corni Officinalis (*Shan Zhu Yu*)
Radix Dioscoreae Oppositae (*Shan Yao*)
Sclerotium Poriae Cocoris (*Fu Ling*)
Radix Praeparatus Glycyrrhizae (*Zhi Gan Cao*)

B. Moistening yin & descending fire

This method of treatment is used for vacuity fire arising from yin vacuity or loss of communication between the heart and kidneys causing turbid *lin* and spermatorrhea. The basic formulas for these include the use of *Gu Jing Wan* and *Zhi Bai Di Huang Wan* plus *Si Yin Jian*.

Gu Jing Wan

Plastrum Testudinis (*Gui Ban*)
Radix Rubrus Paeoniae Lactiflorae (*Chi Shao*)
Radix Scutellariae Baicalensis (*Huang Qin*)
Cortex Phellodendri (*Huang Bai*)
Cortex Cedrelae (*Chun Bai*)
Rhizoma Cyperi Rotundi (*Xiang Fu*)

Zhi Bai Di Huang Wan

Rhizoma Anemarrhenae (*Zhi Mu*)
Cortex Phellodendri (*Huang Bai*)
Radix Coquitus Rehmanniae (*Shu Di*)
Fructus Corni Officinalis (*Shan Zhu Yu*)

Radix Dioscoreae Oppositae (*Shan Yao*)
Sclerotium Poriae Cocoris (*Fu Ling*)
Cortex Radicis Moutan (*Dan Pi*)
Rhizoma Alismatis (*Ze Xie*)

Si Yin Jian

Radix Rehmanniae (*Sheng Di*), 12g
Tuber Ophiopogonis Japonicae (*Mai Dong*), 10g
Radix Albus Paeoniae Lactiflorae (*Bai Shao*), 10g
Bulbus Lilii (*Bai He*), 9g
Radix Glehniae Littoralis (*Sha Shen*), 18g
Radix Glycyrrhizae (*Sheng Gan Cao*), 3g
Sclerotium Poriae Cocoris (*Fu Ling*), 9g

C. Supplementing the kidneys & clearing heat

Excess heat exhausting the body fluids and yin may cause *lin* symptoms, incontinence of urine, painful urination, and bloody semen. The basic formula used is *Hua Yin Jian*.

Hua Yin Jian

Radix Rehmanniae (*Sheng Di*), 10g
Radix Coquitus Rehmanniae (*Shu Di*), 10g
Radix Achyranthis Bidentatae (*Niu Xi*), 10g
Sclerotium Polypori Umbellati (*Zhu Ling*), 10g
Rhizoma Alismatis (*Ze Xie*), 10g
Cortex Phellodendri (*Huang Bai*), 10g
Rhizoma Anemarrhenae (*Zhi Mu*), 10g
Semen Phaseoli Radiati (*Lu Dou*), 12g
Radix Gentianae Scabrae (*Long Dan Cao*), 8g
Semen Plantaginis (*Che Qian Zi*), 6g

D. Warming & consolidating the kidneys

Vacuity of the kidneys and lower burner may result in turbid *lin* and spermatorrhea. The appropriate formula is *You Gui Yin*.

You Gui Yin

Radix Coquitus Rehmanniae (*Shu Di*)
Radix Praeparatus Aconiti Carmichaeli (*Fu Zi*)
Cortex Cinnamomi (*Rou Gui*)
Fructus Corni Officinalis (*Shan Zhu Yu*)
Fructus Lycii Chinensis (*Gou Qi Zi*)
Radix Dioscoreae Oppositae (*Shan Yao*)
Cortex Eucommiae Ulmoidis (*Du Zhong*)
Radix Praeparatus Glycyrrhizae (*Zhi Gan Cao*)

E. Warming the kidneys & strengthening yang

Exhaustion of the *ming men*, *jing qi* vacuity, and cold can cause impotence, premature ejaculation, and sterility. The appropriate formula is *Zang Yu Dan*.

Zan Yu Dan

Radix Coquitus Rehmanniae (*Shu Di*)
Rhizoma Atractylodis Macrocephalae (*Bai Zhu*)
Radix Angelicae Sinensis (*Dang Gui*)
Fructus Lycii Chinensis (*Gou Qi*)
Cortex Eucommiae Ulmoidis (*Du Zhong*)
Rhizoma Curculiginis Orchoidis (*Xian Mao*)
Fructus Corni Officinalis (*Shan Zhu Yu*)
Herba Epimedii (*Yin Yang Huo*)
Herba Cistanchis (*Rou Cong Rong*)
Semen Allii Tuberosi (*Jiu Cai Zi*)
Semen Cnidii Monnieri (*She Chuang Zi*)
Radix Praeparatus Aconiti Carmichaeli (*Fu Zi*)
Cortex Cinnamomi (*Rou Gui*)
Radix Morindae Officinalis (*Ba Ji Tian*)

2. Activating the blood & transforming stasis

Stasis is a common element in male urological disorders including variocele, failure to ejaculate due to obstruction of the spermatic chord, impotence, uncontrollable erection, bloody semen, thickened semen, penile tumor, orchioneus, epididymal carcinoma, orchioscrotal cancer, chronic prostatitis, prostamegaly, etc. Treatment of these conditions should be based on pattern discrimination. This means that one should determine what is stagnant and static and to what degree before choosing a formula or medicinals. Two commonly used formulas for activating the blood and transforming stasis are *Xue Fu Zhu Yu Tang* and *Yi Wei Dan Shen Yin*.

Xue Fu Zhu Yu Tang

Radix Angelicae Sinensis (*Dang Gui*), 9g
Radix Rehmanniae (*Sheng Di*), 9g
Flos Carthami Tinctorii (*Hong Hua*), 9g
Radix Achyranthis Bidentatae (*Huai Niu Xi*), 9g
Semen Pruni Persicae (*Tao Ren*), 12g
Fructus Citri Seu Ponciri (*Zhi Ke*), 6g
Radix Rubrus Paeoniae Lactiflorae (*Chi Shao*), 6g
Radix Bupleuri (*Chai Hu*), 3g
Raix Glycyrrhizae (*Gan Cao*), 3g
Radix Platycodi Grandiflori (*Jie Geng*), 4.5g
Rhizoma Ligustici Wallichii (*Chuan Xiong*), 4.5g

Yi Wei Dan Shen Yin

Radix Salviae Miltiorrhizae (*Dan Shen*), 12g

3. Transforming phlegm & dispelling stasis

Urological disorders, such as impotence, spermatorrhea with or without dreams, failure to ejaculate, and prostamegaly, may be due to lingering phlegm and stasis, and especially in chronic disorders.

In this case, one should transform phlegm and dispel stasis. One common formula which transforms phlegm and dispels stasis is *Qing Qi Hua Tan Wan*.

Qing Qi Hua Tan Wan

Semen Trichosanthis Kirlowii (*Gua Lou Ren*)
Radix Scutellariae Baicalensis (*Huang Qin*)
Pericarpium Citri Erythrocarpae (*Ju Hong*)
Semen Pruni Armeniacae (*Xing Ren*)
Fructus Immaturus Citri Seu Ponciri (*Zhi Shi*)
Sclerotium Poriae Cocoris (*Fu Ling*)
Rhizoma Praeparata Cum Fellem Bovim Arisaematis (*Dan Nan Xing*)
Rhizoma Pinelliae Ternatae (*Ban Xia*)

4. Treating liver disorders

One of the main internal organs involved in male urology is the liver. In liver related disorders, the liver may need to be drained, warmed, dispersed, softened, or even supplemented. Each of these is a different principle or method of treating the liver and different guiding formulas and medicinals must be selected to accomplish each of these ends. Thus it is extremely important when treating liver disorders to correctly discriminate the extact pattern of disharmony involved. Two formulas used to treat liver disorders causing urological disease are *Da Yi Tang* and *Kai Yu Zhong Zi Tang*.

Da Yi Tang

Rhizoma Cimicifugae (*Sheng Ma*)
Radix Bupleuri (*Chai Hu*)
Rhizoma Ligustici Wallichii (*Chuan Xiong*)
Rhizoma Cyperi Rotundi (*Xiang Fu*)
Semen Tribuli Terrestris (*Bai Ji Li*)
Cortex Radicis Mori (*Sang Bai Pi*)

Folium Citri Reticulatae (*Ju Ye*)

Kai Yu Zhong Yu Tang

Radix Albus Paeoniae Lactiflorae (*Bai Shao*)
Rhizoma Cyperi Rotundi (*Xiang Fu*)
Radix Angelicae Sinensis (*Dang Gui*)
Rhizoma Atractylodis Macrocephalae (*Bai Zhu*)
Cortex Radicis Moutan (*Dan Pi*)
Sclerotium Poriae Cocoris (*Fu Ling*)
Radix Trichosanthis Kirlowii (*Tian Hua Fen*)

5. Treating the *jing*

The *jing* is the root of male sexual function. Many sexual dysfunction diseases involve the *jing* according to TCM theory. The *jing* may be disordered in a variety of ways and, therefore, there is more than one treatment method which addresses *jing* disorders. The TCM treatment methods which address the *jing* are:

A. Boosting the qi and generating *jing*.

These methods are used for the treatment of *jing qi* vacuity. The following medicinals accomplish these ends:

Radix Codonopsis Pilosulae (*Dang Shen*)
Radix Astragali Seu Hedysari (*Huang Qi*)
Radix Praeparatus Aconiti Carmichaeli (*Fu Zi*)
Cornu Degelatinum Cervi (*Lu Jiao Shuang*)
Radix Morindae Officinalis (*Ba Ji Tian*)
Radix Dioscoreae Oppositae (*Shan Yao*)

B. Nourishing the blood and generating *jing*.

These methods are used for blood vacuity and *jing* exhaustion. The following medicinals accomplish these ends:

Radix Angelicae Sinensis (*Dang Gui*)
Radix Coquitus Rehmanniae (*Shu Di*)
Radix Polygoni Multiflori (*He Shou Wu*)
Radix Albus Paeoniae Lactiflorae (*Bai Shao*)
Gelatinum Corii Asini (*E Jiao*)
Colla Cornu Cervi (*Lu Jiao Jiao*)
Caulis Milletiae Seu Spatholobi (*Ji Xue Teng*)
Fructus Lycii Chinensis (*Gou Qi Zi*)
Placenta Hominis (*Zi He Che*)

C. Supplementing the kidneys and replenishing the *jing*.

If kidney *jing* exhaustion with yang vacuity predominates, the following medicinals accomplish these ends:

Radix Praeparatus Aconiti Carmichaeli (*Fu Zi*)
Cortex Cinnamomi (*Rou Gui*)
Cornu Cervi Parvum (*Lu Rong*)
Radix Morindae Officinalis (*Ba Ji Tian*)
Rhizoma Curculiginis Orchoidis (*Xian Mao*)
Herba Epimedii (*Xian Ling Pi*)
Semen Trigonellae Foeni-graeci (*Hu Lu Bao*)
Semen Astragali (*Sha Yuan Zi*)
Testes Canitis (*Guang Gou Shen*)
Herba Cynomorii Songarici (*Suo Yang*)
Herba Cistanchis (*Rou Cong Rong*)
Fructus Psoraleae Corylifoliae (*Bu Gu Zhi*)

If kidney *jing* exhaustion with yin vacuity predominates, the following medicinals accomplish these ends:

Fructus Ligustri Lucidi (*Nu Zhen Zi*)
Herba Ecliptae Prostratae (*Han Lian Cao*)
Fructus Mori Albi (*Sang Shen Zi*)
Fructus Lycii Chinensis (*Gou Qi*)
Fructus Corni Officinalis (*Shan Yu Rou*)

Plastrum Testudinis (*Gui Ban*)
Carapax Amydae (*Bie Jia*)

D. Astringing the qi & consolidating the *jing*

The following medicinals accomplish these ends:

Radix Astragali Seu Hedysari (*Huang Qi*)
Radix Codonopsis Pilosulae (*Dang Shen*)
Rhizoma Atractylodis Macrocephalae (*Bai Zhu*)
Semen Euryalis Ferocis (*Qian Shi*)
Semen Nelumbinis Nuciferae (*Lian Shi*)
Radix Dioscoreae Oppositae (*Shan Yao*)
Radix Albus Paeoniae Lactiflorae (*Bai Shao*)
Fructus Schizandrae Chinensis (*Wu Wei Zi*)
Galla Rhi Chinensis (*Wu Bei Zi*)
Os Calcinatus Draconis (*Duan Long Gu*)
Concha Calcinata Ostreae (*Duan Mu Li*)
Fructus Corni Officinalis (*Shan Yu Rou*)
Ootheca Mantidis (*Sang Piao Xiao*)

E. Boosting the kidneys & consolidating the *jing*

These treatment methods are used in cases of spermatorrhea due
to kidney vacuity. The following medicinals accomplish these ends:

Fructus Corni Officinalis (*Shan Yu Rou*)
Fructus Lycii Chinensis (*Gou Qi*)
Galla Rhi Chinensis (*Wu Bei Zi*)
Semen Euryalis Ferocis (*Qian Shi*)
Fructus Psoraleae Corylifoliae (*Bu Gu Zhi*)
Rhizoma Curculiginis Orchoidis (*Xian Mao*)
Herba Epimedii (*Xian Ling Pi*)
Semen Cnidii Monnieri (*She Chuang Zi*)
Os Carbonisatus Draconis (*Duan Long Gu*)
Concha Calcinata Ostreae (*Duan Mu Li*)

F. Resolving toxins & increasing *jing*

These treatment methods are used together in cases of damp heat injuring the *jing* essence. The following medicinals accomplish these ends:

Herba Polygoni Avicularis (*Bian Xu*)
Herba Cum Radice Taraxaci Mongolici (*Pu Gong Ying*)
Herba Oldenlandiae Diffusae (*Bai Hua She She Cao*)
Semen Coicis Lachryma-jobi (*Yi Yi Ren*)
Flos Lonicerae Japonicae (*Yin Hua*)

G. Stopping bleeding & boosting the *jing*

These treatment methods are used together for pouring down of blood and *jing*. The following medicinals accomplish these ends:

Radix Carbonisatus Rehmanniae (*Sheng Di Tan*)
Flos Carbonisatus Lonicerae Japonicae (*Yin Hua Tan*)
Pollen Carbonisatus Typhae (*Pu Huang Tan*)
Crinis Carbonisatus (*Xue Yu*)
Nodus Carbonisatus Rhizomatis Nelumbinis Nuciferae (*Ou Jie Tan*)
Cortex Carbonisatus Eucommiae Ulmoidis (*Du Zhong Tan*)

H. Activating the blood & freeing the flow of *jing*

These methods are used to treat *jing yu zheng* or *jing* stasis pathocondition. One formula appropriate for accomplishing these ends is composed of:

Apex Radicis Angelicae Sinensis (*Dang Gui Wei*)
Caulis Milletiae Seu Spatholobi (*Ji Xue Teng*)
Herba Leonuri Heterophylli (*Yi Mu Cao*)
Radix Achyranthis Bidentatae (*Niu Xi*)
Flos Carthami Tinctorii (*Hong Hua*)
Squama Manitis (*Chuan Shan Jia*)

Semen Vaccariae Segetalis (*Wang Bu Liu Xing*)
Radix Pseudoginseng (*San Qi*)

I. Descending the qi & returning the *jing*

These methods are used to treat retroversion of the flow of sperm
into the bladder. One formula appropriate for accomplishing these
ends is composed of:

Lignum Aquilariae Agallochae (*Chen Xiang*)
Lignum Dalbergiae Odoriferae (*Jiang Xiang*)
Semen Litchi Chinensis (*Li Zhi He*)
Magnetitum (*Ci Shi*)
Radix Linderae Strychnifoliae (*Wu Yao*)
Semen Cnidii Monnieri (*She Chuang Zi*)

J. Depressing yang & assisting yin

These methods are used to treat yang repletion and yin vacuity.
One formula appropriate for accomplishing these ends is
composed of:

Fructus Ligustri Lucidi (*Nu Zhen Zi*)
Radix Polygoni Multiflori (*He Shou Wu*)
Fructus Mori Albi (*Sang Shen Zi*)
Rhizoma Anemarrhenae (*Zhi Mu*)
Cortex Phellodendri (*Huang Bai*)
Plastrum Testudinis (*Gui Ban*)

Commonly used prescriptions in China for the treatment of urological disorders

1. *Long Dan Xie Gan Tang*

Radix Gentianae Scabrae (*Long Dan Cao*)
Radix Scutellariae Baicalensis (*Huang Qin*)

Fructus Gardeniae Jasminoidis (*Zhi Zi*)
Rhizoma Alismatis (*Ze Xie*)
Semen Plantaginis (*Che Qian Zi*)
Caulis Akebiae Mutong (*Mu Tong*)
Radix Rehmanniae (*Sheng Di*)
Apex Radicis Angelicae Sinensis (*Dang Gui Wei*)
Radix Bupleuri (*Chai Hu*)
Radix Glycyrrhizae (*Gan Cao*)

This formula is used to clear heat and disinhibit dampness and to discharge true fire from the liver channel. It is especially apropriate for treating replete fire going upward, with damp heat pouring downward in the liver channel. In urology, this formula is used to treat swelling of the external genitalia, impotence, spermatorrhea, bloody semen, persistent erection, failure to ejaculate, etc. due to liver channel damp heat pouring downward.

2. *Shao Fu Zhu Yu Tang*

Radix Angelicae Sinensis (*Dang Gui*)
Rhizoma Ligustici Wallichii (*Chuan Xiong*)
Radix Rubrus Paeoniae Lactiflorae (*Chi Shao*)
Fructus Foeniculi Vulgaris (*Xiao Hui Xiang*)
Rhizoma Corydalis Yanhusuo (*Yuan Hu*)
Feces Trogopterori Seu Pteromi (*Wu Ling Zhi*)
Myrrha (*Mo Yao*)
Cortex Cinnamomi (*Rou Gui*)
Rhizoma Desiccata Zingiberis (*Gan Jiang*)
Pollen Typhae (*Pu Huang)*

This formula warms the channels, dispels cold, and transforms stasis. It is, therefore, used for conditions characterized as cold stagnation with blood stasis. In urology, this prescription is used to treat pain of the testes during copulation, failure to ejaculate, lack of sperm, impotence, bloody sperm, atrophy of the penis, etc.

3. *Wu Zi Heng Zhong Wan*

Fructus Lycii Chinensis (*Gou Qi Zi*)
Semen Cuscutae (*Tu Si Zi*)
Fructus Schizandrae Chinensis (*Wu Wei Zi*)
Fructus Rubi (*Fu Pen Zi*)
Semen Plantaginis (*Che Qian Zi*)

This formula supplements the kidneys and boosts the *jing*. Therefore, it is used to treat kidney *jing* vacuity conditions. In urology, it is used for impotence, decreased sexual function, failure to ejaculate, spermatorrhea, maldevelopment of the sperm, dead sperm, lack of semen, etc.

4. *Zhi Bai Di Huang Wan*

Rhizoma Anemarrhenae (*Zhi Mu*)
Cortex Phellodendri (*Huang Bai*)
Radix Coquitus Rehmanniae (*Shu Di*)
Fructus Corni Officinalis (*Shan Yu Rou*)
Radix Dioscoreae Oppositae (*Shan Yao*)
Cortex Radicis Moutan (*Dan Pi*)
Rhizoma Alismatis (*Ze Xie*)
Sclerotium Poriae Cocoris (*Fu Ling*)

This formula moistens yin and descends fire. It is indicated for the treatment of yin vacuity with stirring of false fire. In urology, it is used to treat premature ejaculation, impotence, spermatorrhea, bloody semen, persistent erection, failure to ejaculate, etc.

5. *Ma Huang Xi Xin Fu Zi Tang*

Herba Ephedra Sinicae (*Ma Huang*)
Radix Praeparatus Aconiti Carmichaeli (*Fu Zi*)
Herba Cum Radice Asari Seiboldi (*Xi Xin*)

This formula warms the channels and assists yang, dispels cold and resolves toxins. It is indicated for the treatment of internal vacuity with attack by external cold evils. In urology, it is used to treat external cold causing yang qi vacuity with blockage of the channels causing impotence and painful penis and testes.

6. Gui Zhi Jia Long Gu Mu Li Tang

Ramulus Cinnamomi (*Gui Zhi*)
Radix Albus Paeoniae Lactiflorae (*Bai Shao*)
Os Draconis (*Long Gu*)
Concha Ostreae (*Mu Li*)
Fructus Zizyphi Jujubae (*Da Zao*)
Radix Glycyrrhizae (*Gan Cao*)

This formula treats imbalances of yin and yang. In urology, it is used to treat failure to ejaculate due to vacuity of heart and kidneys, impotence, premature ejaculation, etc.

7. San Ren Tang

Semen Pruni Armeniacae (*Xing Ren*)
Fructus Amomi Cardamomi (*Bai Dou Kou*)
Cortex Magnoliae Officinalis (*Hou Po*)
Rhizoma Pinelliae Ternatae (*Ban Xia*)
Semen Coicis Lachryma-jobi (*Yi Yi Ren*)
Medulla Tetrapanacis Papyriferi (*Tong Cao*)
Herba Lophatheri Gracilis (*Dan Zhu Ye*)
Talcum (*Hua Shi*)

This formula courses and regulates the qi mechanism, clears heat, and transforms dampness. In urology, it is used for treating spermatorrhea, impotence, premature ejaculation, failure to ejaculate, sterility, and hernia or water *shan*.

Commonly used prescriptions for urological disorders in Japan

These formulas are some of the most commonly used Chinese

formulas used in Japan for the treatment of male urological and sexual dysfunction disorders. Their use in a given disease should depend upon the patient's pattern discrimination diagnosis.

Japanese *kanpo yaku* or Chinese herbal medicine is mostly based on pre-Jin/Yuan Dynasty formulas. These formulas are composed of typically fewer ingredients than modern Chinese TCM formulas and their ingredients are relatively cheap and commonplace. In addition, these formulas are widely available in the West as both desiccated, powdered extracts and pills. Therefore, their use in the West is not dependent upon access to a Chinese apothecary.

Further, practitioners of *kanpo yaku* do not seem to modify formulas as much as modern Chinese practitioners. Although results may not be as quick and dramatic using these *gu fang* or ancient formulas, they are appropriate for use by beginners, in which case speed of cure is counterbalanced by simplicity and ease of both prescription and administration. However, the practitioner and patient should both be aware that patience may be required. This is not inappropriate in the treatment of chronic diseases. Since the majority of male urological disease tend to manifest after 40 years of age, most male urological diseases are, in fact, chronic, deep-seated conditions.

Acute prostatitis

1. *Da Huang Mu Dan Pi Tang*

Radix Et Rhizoma Rhei (*Da Huang*)
Cortex Radicis Moutan (*Dan Pi*)
Semen Benincasae Hispidae (*Dong Gua Ren*)
Mirabilitum (*Mang Xiao*)
Semen Pruni Persicae (*Tao Ren*)

2. *Long Dan Xie Gan Tang* (see above)

3. *Wu Ling San*

Sclerotium Polypori Umbellati (*Zhu Ling*)
Sclerotium Poriae Cocoris (*Fu Ling*)
Rhizoma Alismatis (*Ze Xie*)
Ramulus Cinnamomi (*Gui Zhi*)
Rhizoma Atractylodis Macrocephalae (*Bai Zhu*)

Testitis

1. *Da Huang Mu Dan Pi Tang* (see above)

2. *Long Dan Xue Gan Tang* (see above)

Chronic prostatitis

1. *Ba Wei Di Huang Wan*

Radix Coquitus Rehmanniae (*Shu Di*)
Fructus Corni Officinalis (*Shan Yu Rou*)
Radix Dioscoreae Oppositae (*Shan Yao*)
Cortex Cinnamomi (*Rou Gui*)
Radix Praeparatus Aconiti Carmichaeli (*Fu Zi*)
Cortex Radicis Moutan (*Dan Pi*)
Rhizoma Alismatis (*Ze Xie*)
Sclerotium Poriae Cocoris (*Fu Ling*)

2. *Wu Ling San* (see above)

3. *Long Dan Xie Gan Tang* (see above)

4. *Qing Xin Lian Zi Yin*

Semen Nelumbinis Nuciferae (*Lian Zi*)
Radix Panacis Ginseng (*Ren Shen*)
Tuber Ophiopogonis Japonicae (*Mai Dong*)
Sclerotium Poriae Cocoris (*Fu Ling*)

Radix Scutellariae Baicalensis (*Huang Qin*)
Radix Astragali Seu Hedysari (*Huang Qi*)
Semen Plantaginis (*Che Qian Zi*)
Cortex Radicis Lycii (*Di Gu Pi*)
Radix Glycyrrhizae (*Gan Cao*)

5. Jia Wei Xiao Yao San

Radix Bupleuri (*Chai Hu*)
Radix Albus Paeoniae Lactiflorae (*Bai Shao*)
Radix Angelicae Sinensis (*Dang Gui*)
Rhizoma Atractylodis Macrocephalae (*Bai Zhu*)
Sclerotium Poriae Cocoris (*Fu Ling*)
Fructus Gardeniae Jasminoidis (*Zhi Zi*)
Cortex Radicis Moutan (*Dan Pi*)
Radix Praeparatus Glycyrrhizae (*Zhi Gan Cao*)
Herba Menthae (*Bo He*)
Rhizoma Recens Zingiberis (*Sheng Jiang*)

Prostatic hypertrophy

1. Da Huang Mu Dan Pi (see above)

2. Long Dan Xie Gan Tang (see above)

3. Wu Ling San (see above)

4. Ba Wei Di Huang Wan (see above)

5. Teng Long Tang

Cortex Radicis Moutan (*Dan Pi*)
Semen Pruni Persicae (*Tao Ren*)
Semen Benincasae Hispidae (*Dong Gua Ren*)
Rhizoma Atractylodis Macrocephalae (*Bai Zhu*)
Semen Coicis Lachryma-jobi (*Yi Yi Ren*)
Radix Et Rhizoma Rhei (*Da Huang*)

Mirabilitum (*Mang Xiao*)
Radix Glycyrrhizae (*Gan Cao*)

6. *Tao He Cheng Qi Tang*

Semen Pruni Persicae (*Tao Ren*)
Radix Et Rhizoma Rhei (*Da Huang*)
Mirabilitum (*Mang Xiao*)
Ramulus Cinnamomi (*Gui Zhi*)
Radix Glycyrrhizae (*Gan Cao*)

Impotence

1. *Ba Wei Di Huang Wan* (see above)

2. *Gui Zhi Jia Long Gu Mu Li Tang* (see above)

3. *Chai Hu Jia Long Gu Mu Li Tang*

Radix Bupleuri (*Chai Hu*)
Os Draconis (*Long Gu*)
Concha Ostreae (*Mu Li*)
Rhizoma Pinelliae Ternatae (*Ban Xia*)
Sclerotium Poriae Cocoris (*Fu Ling*)
Ramulus Cinnamomi (*Gui Zhi*)
Radix Scutellariae Baicalensis (*Huang Qin*)
Radix Panacis Ginseng (*Ren Shen*)
Radix Et Rhizoma Rhei (*Da Huang*)
Fructus Zizyphi Jujubae (*Da Zao*)
Rhizoma Recens Zingiberis (*Sheng Jiang*)

4. *Xiao Chai Hu Tang*

Radix Bupleuri (*Chai Hu*)
Radix Scutellariae Baicalensis (*Huang Qin*)
Rhizoma Pinelliae Ternatae (*Ban Xia*)
Radix Codonopsis Pilosulae (*Dang Shen*)

Fructus Zizyphi Jujubae (*Da Zao*)
Rhizoma Recens Zingiberis (*Sheng Jiang*)
Radix Praeparatus Glycyrrhizae (*Zhi Gan Cao*)

Scrotal edema

1. *Fang Ji Huang Qi Tang*

Radix Stephaniae Tetrandrae (*Han Fang Ji*)
Radix Astragali Seu Hedysari (*Huang Qi*)
Rhizoma Atractylodis Macrocephalae (*Bai Zhu*)
Fructus Zizyphi Jujubae (*Da Zao*)
Rhizoma Recens Zingiberis (*Sheng Jiang*)
Radix Glycyrrhizae (*Gan Cao*)

2. *Wu Lin San Jia Wei*

Sclerotium Poriae Cocoris (*Fu Ling*)
Radix Angelicae Sinensis (*Dang Gui*)
Radix Albus Paeoniae Lactiflorae (*Bai Shao*)
Fructus Gardeniae Jasminoidis (*Zhi Zi*)
Radix Glycyrrhizae (*Gan Cao*)
Semen Plantaginis (*Che Qian Zi*)
Caulis Akebiae Mutong (*Mu Tong*)

3. *Ban Xia Hou Po Tang*

Cortex Magnoliae Officinalis (*Hou Po*)
Rhizoma Pinelliae Ternatae (*Ban Xia*)
Sclerotium Poriae Cocoris (*Fu Ling*)
Fructus Perillae Frutescentis (*Su Zi*)
Rhizoma Recens Zingiberis (*Sheng Jiang*)

4. *Long Dan Xie Gan Tang* (see above)

Difficulty in sexual function

1. *Gui Zhi Jia Long Gu Mu Li Tang* (see above)

2. *Ba Wei Di Huang Wan* (see above)

3. *Chai Hu Jia Long Gu Mu Li Tang* (see above)

4. *Da Chai Hu Tang*

Radix Bupleuri (*Chai Hu*)
Radix Et Rhizoma Rhei (*Da Huang*)
Radix Scutellariae Baicalensis (*Huang Qin*)
Rhizoma Pinelliae Ternatae (*Ban Xia*)
Fructus Immaturus Citri Seu Ponciri (*Zhi Shi*)
Radix Albus Paeoniae Lactiflorae (*Bai Shao*)
Fructus Zizyphi Jujubae (*Da Zao*)
Rhizoma Recens Zingiberis (*Sheng Jiang*)

5. *Gui Zhi Jia Fu Zi Tang*

Ramulus Cinnamomi (*Gui Zhi*)
Radix Albus Paeoniae Lactiflorae (*Bai Shao*)
Radix Praeparatus Aconiti Carmichaeli (*Fu Zi*)
Fructus Zizyphi Jujubae (*Da Zao*)
Rhizoma Desiccata Zingiberis (*Gan Jiang*)
Radix Glycyrrhizae (*Gan Cao*)

6. *Dang Gui Si Ni Tang*

Radix Angelicae Sinensis (*Dang Gui*)
Ramulus Cinnamomi (*Gui Zhi*)
Radix Albus Paeoniae Lactiflorae (*Bai Shao*)
Caulis Akebiae Mutong (*Mu Tong*)
Herba Cum Radice Asari Seiboldi (*Xi Xin*)
Fructus Zizyphi Jujubae (*Da Zao*)
Radix Praeparatus Glycyrrhizae (*Zhi Gan Cao*)

7. *Wu Zhu Yu Tang*

Fructus Evodiae Rutecarpae (*Wu Zhu Yu*)
Radix Panacis Ginseng (*Ren Shen*)
Rhizoma Recens Zingiberis (*Sheng Jiang*)
Fructus Zizyphi Jujubae (*Da Zao*)

8. *Yi Gan San Jia Bai Shao Tang*

Radix Bupleuri (*Chai Hu*)
Radix Angelicae Sinensis (*Dang Gui*)
Radix Albus Paeoniae Lactiflorae (*Bai Shao*)
Rhizoma Ligustici Wallichii (*Chuan Xiong*)
Ramulus Uncariae Cum Uncis (*Gou Teng*)
Sclerotium Poriae Cocoris (*Fu Ling*)
Rhizoma Atractylodis Macrocephalae (*Bai Zhu*)
Radix Glycyrrhizae (*Gan Cao*)

Sterility

1. *Ba Wei Di Huang Wan* (see above)

2. *Bu Zhong Yi Qi Tang*

Radix Codonopsis Pilosulae (*Dang Shen*)
Radix Astragali Seu Hedysari (*Huang Qi*)
Rhizoma Atractylodis Macrocephalae (*Bai Zhu*)
Radix Angelicae Sinensis (*Dang Gui*)
Radix Bupleuri (*Chai Hu*)
Rhizoma Cimicifugae (*Sheng Ma*)
Pericarpium Citri Reticulatae (*Chen Pi*)
Radix Praeparatus Glycyrrhizae (*Zhi Gan Cao*)

These two formulas can also be used together.

3. Ren Shen Tang

Radix Panacis Ginseng (*Ren Shen*)
Rhizoma Atractylodis Macrocephalae (*Bai Zhu*)
Radix Praeparatus Glycyrrhizae (*Zhi Gan Cao*)
Rhizoma Recens Zingiberis (*Sheng Jiang*)

This formula can also be combined with *Ba Wei Di Huang Wan*.

8

Dietary Therapy for Sexual Dysfunction

As stated above, the kidneys store the two types of *jing*, namely congenital *jing* and acquired essence. The sexual function of the healthy person depends upon these two types of *jing*. A healthy diet provides adequate nutrients to support the *zang fu zhi jing* or the essence of the organs and bowels, and this can greatly support sexual function. In Traditional Chinese Medicine, in order to maintain the body's health, medicinal supplementation should be coupled with proper diet. Thus there is the saying, "7 parts dietary therapy, 3 parts herbal treatment."

Balancing one's food intake as the key to a healthy diet

A balanced intake of food can help establish and maintain a healthy balance between yin and yang and enrich the *jing* and blood. This may then improve sexual function and remedially benefit the recovery from sexual dysfunction. Balancing one's food intake implies eating grains as one's main food or staple, supplemented by vegetables and meats. Insufficient intake in any of these three groups of food may result in deficiencies of yin or yang, qi or blood, and premature aging.

Depending on their nature and flavor, different foods have different effects on the body's metabolism. Therefore, different foods are used to treat different patients and different diseases. These differences are all likewise predicated on a TCM *bian zheng* diagnosis. For instance, cool and cold foods can help clear heat and purge fire from the body, whereas, sweet and cold foods can help moisten yin and descend fire as well as generate body fluids. Warm and hot foods warm the yang and supplement insufficiency, while sweet and warm foods warm the *ming men* and boost yang qi. Thus each food should be decided upon based on its nature and temperature in realtionship to the pattern of the patient being treated.

Lamb and shrimp are the best foods for treating kidney yang vacuity and weakness of *ming men* fire. Sweet, cold, and salty foods, such as Carapax Amydae (*Bie Jia*) and Concha Ostreae (*Mu Li*), moisten yin and descend fire in the treatment of dysfunctions due to yin vacuity and effulgent fire with loss of communication between the heart and kidneys. Sweet, salty, warm foods, such as seaweed and fish, can replenish essence and supplement the blood in essence blood vacuities. Cool, bitter, sweet, and salty foods, such as bitter melon and winter melon, are used to clear heat and disinhibit dampness in the treatment of damp heat dirsorders. Thus the different natures and flavors of different foods should be studied carefully to help maintain the balance of yin and yang throughout one's life.

Additionally, different foods should be eaten in different seasons. Patients with sexual dysfunction should eat supplementing foods in the spring. They should eat sweet, bitter, and cool foods in the summer, such as mung beans, lotus, watermelon, bitter melon, etc. These can clear heat and disinhibit dampness due to their bitter, sweet, cold nature. Autumn is a dry season; therefore, it is best to eat cooling, moistening foods, such as Radix Glehniae Littoralis (*Sha Shen*), Semen Sesami Indici (*Zi Ma*), and cane sugar to clear the qi and moisten dryness. And during the cold season of winter, pungent, sweet, warm or hot foods, such as dog meat, Cornu Cervi Parvum (*Lu Rong*), and jujubes, are appropriate since they can help warm and supplement the spleen and kidneys, boost the qi, and replenish the essence.

Foods for increasing sexual function

Most sexual dysfunctions are rooted in vacuity conditions and especially chronic deficiencies of the body. Chronic deficiency weaknesses result in an imbalance of yin and yang, which eventually exhausts the *jing* and blood. Disorders of this type are categorized as vacuity patterns, and their principle treatment is to supplement the righteous qi. On the other hand, some patients suffer from damp heat pouring or percolating downward with frenetic or reckless movement of ministerial fire. Thus, both prevention and remedial treatment through dietary therapy should be based on the discrimination of patterns or *bian zheng lun zhi*.

1. Supplementing the kidneys & replenishing the *jing*

Traditionally, Chinese believe that animal products are the best foods for replenishing the *jing*. This includes deer meat and penis, turtle, pig heart and liver, pig brain, lamb liver, heart, and bone amongst others. Food such as this supplement the kidneys, help replenish the *jing*, and benefit the bone marrow. Animal organs such as the kidneys may also be used to supplement the kidney qi, benefit the marrow, and help treat *xu la* diseases. This refers to vacuity taxation or consumptive diseases. In this case, the underlying theory is to, "use the organ to treat that organ's disease." For spermatorrhea due to kidney qi vacuity failing to consolidate the *jing*, one may eat walnuts and pigeon eggs.

2. Warming the kidneys & strengthening yang

Kidney yang vacuity and descension of *ming men* fire manifest as such disorders as decreased sexual drive, impotence, spermatorrhea, premature ejaculation, and cold *jing* causing sterility. Warm foods are indicated for the treatment of such disorders in order to warm kidney yang. Examples of foods which warm kidney yang are lamb, deer meat, and shrimp. These foods are warm in nature and help boost *yuan yang*. Hence they supplement and strengthen the body.

3. Boosting the qi & nourishing the blood

A healthy reproductive system is dependent upon sufficiency of qi
and blood. Any insufficiency of these may result in decreased
libido, impotence, and sterility. To enhance sexual function, it is
therefore necessary to boost the qi and nourish the blood. A few
of the foods which accomplish this are milk, black tree ears,
jujubes, lotus seeds, Gelatinum Corii Asini (*E Jiao*), honey, Radix
Glehniae Littoralis (*Sha Shen*), and grapes.

Foods & medicinals for the remedial treatment
of sexual dysfunction

1. Warming kidney yang

Hippocampus (*Hai Ma*), deer meat, deer penis, lamb, beef, dog
meat, shrimp, walnut

2. Warming the kidneys & replenishing the *jing*

Placenta Hominis (*Zi He Che*), fish abdomen (*Yu Du*), Testis Et
Penis Phocae (*Hai Gou Shen*), Cordyceps Sinensis (*Dong Chong
Xia Cao*), Gecko (*Ge Jie*), pigeon

3. Moistening the kidneys & replenishing the *jing*

Turtle, Concha Ostreae (*Mu Li*), Radix Glehniae Littoralis (*Sha
Shen*), beef marrow, pig marrow

4. Boosting the qi & nourishing the blood

Chicken, Arillus Euphoriae Longanae (*Long Yan Rou*), Fructus
Litchi Chinensis (*Li Zhi*), Radix Dioscoreae Oppositae (*Shan Yao*)

5. Consolidating the kidneys & astringing the essence

Semen Nelumbinis Nuciferae (*Lian Zi*), Plumula Nelumbinis

Nuciferae (*Lian Zi Xin*), whole lotus, (*Lian*), Semen Euryalis Ferocis (*Qian Shi*), Semen Gingkonis Bilobae (*Bai Guo*)

6. Clearing heat & disinhibiting dampness

Winter melon (*Dong Gua*), bitter melon (*Ku Gua*), Plumula Nelumbinis Nuciferae (*Lian Zi Xin*), towel gourd (*Si Gua*)

The flavor, temperature, functions, & indications of the most important foods for increasing male sexual function

Hippocampus (*Hai Ma*)

Nature & flavor: Sweet, salty, & warm

Functions: Supplements kidney yang, regulates the qi and blood

Indications: Impotence, urinary incontinence, and sterlity due to kidney vacuity, vacuity asthma

Deer meat (*Lu Rou*)

Nature & flavor: Sweet & warm

Functions: Warms kidney yang, supplements the spleen and boosts the qi

Indications: Weakness of the lumbar region and knees, impotence, spermatorrhea with or without dreams, and premature ejaculation due to kidney vacuity or vacuity cold, cold scrotum sterility, dizziness and tinnitus

Deer penis (*Lu Bian*)

Nature & flavor: Sweet, salty, & warm

Functions: Supplements the kidneys, strengthens yang, benefits the *jing*

Indications: Weakness and soreness in the low back and knees, and impotence due to kidney qi vacuity, *jing* vacuity sterility

Lamb (*Yang Rou*)

Nature & flavor: Sweet & warm

Functions: Warms the kidneys, strengthens yang, supplements and boosts the qi and blood

Indications: Lumbar pain due to kidney vacuity, impotence and exhausted *jing*, aversion to cold with cold limbs

Beef (*Niu Rou*)

Nature & flavor: Sweet & warm

Functions: Warms and supplements the spleen & kidneys, nourishes the blood and strengthens the sinews

Indications: Impotence, decreased appetite, sighing, weakness and soreness of the lumbar region due to spleen kidney vacuity cold

Dog meat (*Gou Rou*)

Nature & flavor: Salty & warm

Functions: Benefits yang action (*i.e.*, copulation), supplements the blood, strengthens the spleen, astringes the lower burner, replenishes the *jing*

Indications: Lumbar pain, impotence, spermatorrhea, cold and painful low back and knees, and frequent urination due to kidney vacuity

Shrimp (*Xia Rou*)

Nature & flavor: Sweet, salty, & warm

Functions: Supplements kidney yang and strengthens the *jing*

Indications: Impotence, spermatorrhea, premature ejaculaton, frequent urination, and urinary incontinence due to kidney vacuity

Fructus Juglandis Regiae (*Hu Tao Ren*)

Nature & flavor: Sweet & warm

Functions: Supplements the kidneys and strengthens the low back, moistens the lungs and stops asthma

Indications: Frequent urination, weakness, soreness, and painful low back and knees due to lower burner vacuity cold and kidney qi vacuity, vacuity taxation cough and asthma

Placenta Hominis (*Zi He Che*)

Nature & flavor: Sweet, salty, & warm

Functions: Warms the kidneys, supplements the *jing*, boosts the qi, and nourishes the blood

Indications: Vacuity taxation conditions, especially qi and blood exhaustion causing steaming bones, emaciation, premature ejaculation, spermatorrhea with dreams, *jing* exhaustion in men, and infertility in women

Testis Et Penis Phocae (*Hai Gou Shen*)

Nature & flavor: Sweet, salty, & warm

Functions: Warms the kidneys, benefits the *jing*, strengthens the brain and marrow, supplements the blood, moistens dryness, dispels dampness, and disinhibits urination

Indications: Exhaustion of both *jing* and blood causing weakness, frequent urination, spermatorrhea with or without dreams, impotence, and weakness of the lumbar region

Cordyceps Sinensis (*Dong Chong Xia Cao*)

Flavor & nature: Sweet & neutral

Functions: Boosts the qi and *jing*, strengthens the lungs and boosts the kidneys, especially supplements the *ming men*

Indications: Impotence, spermatorrhea, cold sperm, or vacuity after prolonged illness

Gecko (*Ge Jie*)

Flavor & nature: Salty, neutral, slightly toxic

Functions: Supplements lung qi, boosts the *jing* and nourishes the blood, stops cough and asthma, supplements yang

Indications: Impotence and frequent urination due to kidney vacuity, sterility due to low sperm count

Pigeon (*Bai Ge*)

Flavor & nature: Salty & neutral

Functions: Supplements kidney *jing*

Indications: General debility after recovery from prolonged illness, vacuity cold in the lower burner, decreased sex drive

Turtle (*Bei Jia Yu*)

Flavor & nature: Sweet, salty, & neutral

Functions: Supplements the *jing* and nourishes the blood, moistens yin, downbears fire

Indications: Impotence, premature ejaculation, spermatorrhea, weakness of the low back and knees, heat in the five centers or hearts, urinary incontinence, and itching of the external genitalia due to yin vacuity

Carapax Amydae (*Bie Jia*)

Flavor & nature: Sweet, salty, & neutral

Functions: Moistens yin, subdues yang

Indications: Spermatorrhea, impotence, and women's menstrual problems due to insufficiency of kidney yin

Concha Ostreae (*Mu Li*)

Flavor & nature: Sweet, salty, & neutral

Functions: Nourishes yin, subdues yang, supplements the middle burner, astringes the *jing* and perspiration

Indications: Chronic disease, disease of the blood phase, day and night perspiration, spermatorrhea, turbid *lin* or strangury condition, *dai xia* or abnormal vaginal discharge, and *beng lou* or avalanche and leakage (uterine bleeding)

Beef marrow (*Niu Sui*)

Flavor & nature: Sweet & warm

Functions: Supplements the kidneys and replenishes the marrow

Indications: Dual exhaustion of *jing* and blood, general weakness, and cold sperm

Pig marrow (*Zhu Sui*)

Flavor & nature: Sweet & cold

Functions: Supplements yin, replenishes *jing*, benefits the marrow and strengthens the sinews

Indications: Kidney vacuity spermatorrhea, sterility

Fructus Mori Albi (*Sang Shen*)

Flavor & nature: Sour, sweet, & slightly cold

Functions: Nourishes the blood, moistens yin, supplements the liver and kidneys

Indications: Yin vacuity dizziness, insomnia, night sweats, spermatorrhea, premature ejaculation, or constipation

Chicken (*Ji Rou*)

Flavor & nature: Sweet & warm

Functions: Warms the middle burner, boosts the qi, replenishes the *jing* and marrow

Indications: Emaciation, loss of appetite, frequent urination, spermatorrhea, premature ejaculation

Arillus Euphoriae Longanae (*Long Yan Rou*)

Flavor & nature: Sweet & neutral

Functions: Supplements the heart & spleen, calms the spirit, and nourishes the blood

Indications: Dual exhaustion of the heart & spleen causing palpitations, insomnia, forgetfulness, perspiration, and spermatorrhea

Fructus Litchi Chinensis (*Li Zhi*)

Flavor & nature: Sweet, sour, & warm

Functions: Supplements the qi and blood, calms the spirit, and generates fluids

Indications: Spleen vacuity diarrhea, incontinence of urine, hernia, swelling and pain of the scrotum, spermatorrhea, impotence, and decreased sexual drive

Radix Dioscoreae Oppositae (*Shan Yao*)

Flavor & nature: Sweet & neutral

Functions: Strengthens the spleen, supplements the lungs, consolidates the kidneys, and boosts the *jing*

Indications: Spleen kidney vacuity weakness and pain of the low back, frequent urination, spermatorrhea, premature ejaculation, and abnormal vaginal discharge

Lotus (*Lian*)

Flavor & nature: Sweet & neutral

Functions: Supplements the middle burner, calms the spirit, stops diarrhea, and consolidates the *jing*

Indications: Irritability, insomnia, chronic diarrhea, low back pain, and spermatorrhea

Semen Gingkonis Bilobae (*Bai Guo*)

Flavor & nature: Sweet, bitter, neutral, & slightly toxic

Functions: Supplements the kidneys, consolidates the lungs, astringes abnormal vaginal discharge

Indications: Urinary incontinence, spermatorrhea, turbid urine

Winter melon (*Dong Gua*)

Flavor & nature: Sweet, neutral, & cool

Functions: Clear heat, disinhibits water, resolves toxins

Indications: Edema due to damp heat, abnormal vaginal discharge, damp scrotum, soft, weak penis, and spermatorrhea

Bitter melon (*Ku Gua*)

Flavor & nature: Sweet, bitter, & cold

Functions: Clears heat and disinhibits the eyes

Indications: Damp heat diarrhea, swollen, painful genitals, and impotence

Towel gourd (*Si Gua*)

Flavor & nature: Sweet, salty, & cold

Functions: Clears heat, transforms phlegm, cools the blood, and resolves toxins ·

Indications: Damp heat in the liver channel causing impotence, spermatorrhea with dreams, premature ejaculation, fever, thirst, restlessness, and bloody *lin* (*xue lin*)

Book Two

The Treatment of Urological & Male Sexual Dysfunction Diseases

1

Jing Yu Zheng & Tan Yu Zheng Essence Stasis & Phlegm Stasis Pathoconditions

Jing yu zheng
Essence stasis pathocondition

Jing yu implies stasis of the *jing* essence. Because congenital or prenatal *jing* and thus qi, blood, and body fluids form the basic foundation of the human body and its life, *jing* stasis leads to a number of pathoconditions collectively known as *jing yu zheng*. *Jing yu zheng* may be caused by masturbation, inflammation, stagnation, trauma, postsurgical effects such as stagnation of the spermatic duct after vasectomy, prostatitis, testicular hypertrophy, or testicular appendage inflammation. *Jing yu zheng* and kidney blood stasis manifest such symptoms as irritability, restlessness, forgetfulness, insomnia, susceptibility to fright, a dark yellow complexion on the cheeks with dark circles around the eyes, and dark lips and mouth. The skin is dry and the gums are lusterless. There is stabbing pain in the lumbar region and fixed pain in the lower abdomen which is aggravated by pressure. There tend to be purple spots on the tongue and the pulse is strong, forceful, deep, and grating/astringent.

Signs & symptoms:

1. Stabbing pain in the lumbar or kidney region, bottoms of the feet, testes, penis, and lower abdomen. There may be occasional swelling and pain of the testes aggravated by resting/sleeping and

ameliorated by moving.

2. If the patient suffers from impotence or premature ejaculation, they may also suffer from erection without stimulation or fail to experience full erection during copulation, or they may ejaculate without sexual stimulation.

3. Ejaculation is not complete and may occur prior to or after copulation.

4. Incontinence or dripping of urine

5. Premature greying of the hair, loss of hair, itching or painful sensations in the hairy areas of the body, *i.e.* eyebrows, pubic region, mustache, etc.

6. Tinnitus, ringing in the ears

7. A stuffy sensation in the head, chest oppression, retardation of response to stimuli, difficulty concentrating, forgetfulness, insomnia

8. Spermatic quality high in viscosity with increased number of deformed and abnormal sperm count

9. Failure to respond to herbal treatment which previously has not addressed stasis as a major part of the pattern diagnosis

10. Grating/astringent pulse with a dark tongue and purple spots or patches

Therapeutic principles: Activate the blood and free the flow of the *jing*

Guiding Formula: *Huo Xue Tong Jing Tang*

Radix Angelicae Sinensis (*Dang Gui*), 10g
Radix Polygoni Multiflori (*He Shou Wu*), 20g

Herba Leonuri Heterophylli (*Yi Mu Cao*), 20g
Caulis Milletiae Seu Spatholobi (*Ji Xue Teng*), 15g
Radix Achryanthis Bidentatae (*Huai Niu Xi*), 15g
Fructus Lycii Chinensis (*Gou Qi*), 15g
Sanguis Draconis (*Xue Jie*), 5g
Rice wine (*Mi Jiu*)

Additions: The following medicinals may be added depending upon the severity of the individual patient's blood stasis, its location, and their presenting signs and symptoms.

Rhizoma Gusuibu (*Gu Sui Bu*)
Radix Dipsaci (*Xu Duan*)
Pollen Typhae (*Pu Huang*)
Feces Trogopterori Seu Pteromi (*Wu Ling Zhi*)
Semen Pruni Persicae (*Tao Ren*)
Flos Carthami Tinctorii (*Hong Hua*)
Eupolyphagae Seu Opisthoplatiae (*Tu Bie Chong*)
Squama Manitis (*Chuan Shan Jia*)
Semen Vaccariae Segetalis (*Wang Bu Liu Xing*)

For patients suffering from qi vacuity, medicinals which supplement the qi should be added. If qi stagnation exists, qi-moving medicinals should be added. If there is blood stasis, add blood-activating medicinals such as the above. If there is blood vacuity, add blood-nourishing medicinals. For phlegm heat, use appropriate medicinals to clear heat and transform phlegm.

Tan yu zheng
Phlegm stasis pathocondition

Phlegm stasis or *tan yu zheng* resulting from phlegm and damp stagnation may be due to two main causes: 1) overconsumption of greasy, spicy foods, thus forming phlegm and dampness, and 2) qi stagnation transforming into phlegm stasis, in turn due to emotional depression. If phlegm stagnates and accumulates in the body over a long period of time, this will cause obstruction of the channels and connecting vessels which may, in turn, result in male sexual and urological dysfunction.

Signs & symptoms:

1. Muttering to oneself in the chronically ill patient

2. Dull spirit, lusterless eyes, darkness around the eyes, and poor eyesight

3. Obesity with poor muscle tone

4. Increased secretions and body odor in the genital and axillary areas

5. Drowsiness, a heavy sensation in the head, and dizziness

6. Chest oppression and fullness in the epigastrium

7. Restlessness, irritability, and depression

8. A sticky tongue coating with a wiry, slippery, deep, forceful pulse

Bian zheng lun zhi
Treatment on the basis of pattern discrimination

Phlegmatic diseases tend to transform into fire and are usually accompanied by qi stagnation and damp stagnation. The selection of herbal medicinals must, therefore, be made on the basis of an individual pattern discrimination diagnosis.

1. *Tan hua huo*
Phlegm transforming into fire

Pathognomic manifestations: Distention of and a painful feeling in the lower abdomen, short, painful, yellow urine, pain or distention of the external genitalia after intercourse, a red tongue with a yellow, slimy coating, and a wiry, slippery pulse

Therapeutic principles: Clear heat and transform phlegm

Guiding formula:

Rhizoma Arisaematis (*Nan Xing*)
Rhizoma Anemarrhenae (*Zhi Mu*)
Cortex Phellodendri (*Huang Bai*)
Cortex Radicis Lycii Chinensis (*Gi Gu Pi*)
Mirabilitum (*Xuan Ming Fen*)
Caulis Bambusae In Taeniis (*Zhu Ru*)
Succus Bambusae (*Zhu Li*)
Rhizoma Coptidis Chinensis (*Huang Lian*)
Herba Lophatheri Gracilis (*Dan Zhu Ye*)

2. *Tan yu*
  Phlegm stasis

Pathognomic manifestations: Difficulty ejaculating, impotence, a slimy tongue coating, and a slippery or deep, wiry, forceful pulse

Therapeutic principles: Transform phlegm and dispel stasis

Guiding formula:

Sclerotium Polypori Umbellati (*Zhu Ling*)
Sclerotium Poriae Cocoris (*Fu Ling*)
Rhizoma Pinelliae Ternatae (*Fa Ban Xia*)
Rhizoma Alismatis (*Ze Xie*)
Rhizoma Dioscoreae Bi Xie (*Bi Xie*)
Bulbus Fritillariae Cirrhosae (*Chuan Bei Mu*)
Semen Pruni Persicae (*Tao Ren*)
Rhizoma Curcumae Zedoariae (*E Zhu*)
Herba Leonuri Heterophylli (*Yi Mu Cao*)

Herba Lycopi Lucidi (*Ze Lan*)
Scolopendra Subspinipes (*Wu Gong*)

3. *Tan shi*
Phlegm dampness

Pathognomic manifestations: Impotence, premature ejaculation, failure to ejaculate, difficult urination, a flabby, moist tongue, and a slippery pulse

Therapeutic principles: Transform phlegm and perfuse dampness

Guiding formula:

Sclerotium Polypori Umbellati (*Zhu Ling*)
Sclerotium Poriae Cocoris (*Fu Ling*)
Rhizoma Alismatis (*Ze Xie*)
Semen Coicis Lachryma-jobi (*Yi Mi*)
Semen Plantaginis (*Che Qian Zi*)
Rhizoma Atractylodis (*Cang Zhu*)
Rhizoma Atractylodis Macrocephalae (*Bai Zhu*)
Rhizoma Pinelliae Ternatae (*Fa Ban Xia*)
Semen Sinapis Albi (*Bai Jie Zi*)
Scolopendra Subspinipes (*Wu Gong*)

4. *Qi zhi tan yu*
Qi stagnation, phlegm stasis

Pathognomic manifestations: Irritability, restlessness, easily angered, difficult ejaculation, painful intercourse, a slimy, yellow tongue coating, and a wiry, slippery pulse

Therapeutic principles: Move the qi and transform phlegm

Guiding formula:

Radix Bupleuri (*Chai Hu*)

Tuber Curcumae (*Yu Jin*)
Rhizoma Cyperi Rotundi (*Xiang Fu*)
Radix Saussureae Seu Vladimiriae (*Mu Xiang*)
Fructus Citri Sacrodactylis (*Fo Shou*)
Fructus Citri Seu Ponciri (*Zhi Ke*)
Fructus Liquidambaris Taiwanianae (*Lu Lu Tong*)

形不足者，溫之以氣，精不足者，補之以味。

"素問·陰陽應象大論"

If the body is feeble, warm with qi;
if the essence is insufficient,
supplement with flavor

2

Jing Bing **Essence Diseases**

In modern TCM *nan ke*, there are two subcategories of essence diseases. The first includes the more traditional Chinese disease categories involving the essence. This is simply referred to as *jing bing* or essence diseases. The second is called *jing ye yi chang*. This means anomalies in the semen. This subcategory includes several modern Western disease categories concerning the semen and sperm. These disease categories directly relate to male fertility issues.

Jing bing
Essence diseases

Yi jing
Spermatorrhea

Spermatorrhea is defined in TCM as ejaculation without copulation. Under normal conditions, a healthy adult may have a lifestyle which does not include sex. In this case, one may experience spermatorrhea up to three times a month without any signs of discomfort or being categorized as a disease. However, in those who are having sex on a regular basis, due to various pathological factors, spermatorrhea may occur once every 3-5 days or even every other day. This is categorized in TCM as an abnormal condition. If severe, the patient may suffer from multiple episodes of spermatorrhea each night, accompanied by dizziness, fatigue, and weakness of the knees and limbs. In general, pathological spermatorrhea may be further subdivided into two types: with and without dreams. With dreams means that the spermatorrhea is accompanied by erotic or sexual dreams. This is called *yi jing* or loss of essence in Chinese. Without dreams means that the spermatorrhea occurs without simultaneously experiencing any sexual or erotic dreams. This is called *hua jing* or slippery essence in Chinese.

Bing yin bing ji
Disease causes, disease mechanisms

Spermatorrhea may be due to kidney vacuity which is incapable of consolidating or securing the *jing*. This may be due to chronic disease, excessive sex, overuse of drugs, age, excessive taxation, or any other etiological factor leading to weakness and debility of kidney qi. Spermatorrhea may also be due to emotional overtaxation. In this case, excessive emotionality may transform into fire which disturbs the heart spirit, and lead to loss of communication between the kidneys and heart. As heart fire flares upward, kidney *jing* is allowed to slip downward. In addition, spermatorrhea may be due to pathologic invasion of the six external evils, such as dampness and heat, or accumulation of phlegm damp stasis. In either of these cases, the *jing* may be pushed outside its normal passageways by the obstruction of these evil qi.

Phlegm and dampness may be generated internally due to faulty diet and lack of exercise. For instance, overeating raw and chilled foods may injure the spleen's function of transporting and transforming body fluids, which may then accumulate and congeal into phlegm and dampness. Or, overeating greasy, spicy foods may give rise to internally generated damp heat. In this case, not only does the dampness obstruct the free flow of the *jing*, but the evil heat makes it flow outside its bounds, similar to heat's effect on the blood, remembering that there exits a strong relationship between the *jing* and the blood.

Primary approaches to treating spermatorrhea

1. *Zhi xin*
Treating the heart

Although *jing* is stored in the kidneys, it is controlled by the heart. The heart stores the *shen*. When the spirit is calm, stability of the qi is assured. When qi is stable, then water, *i.e.*, the kidneys, is calm, and thus the *jing* is safely housed within the kidneys. Disturbances of the heart, on the other hand, result in restlessness of the spirit. As fire stirs upward, the *shen* may become agitated and, as a result, the patient may suffer from strange dreams and loss of semen during erotic dreams. In addition, the heart generates the blood. Because *jing* and blood share a common source, insufficiency of heart blood may result in kidney *jing* vacuity.

In this case, treatment aimed at supplementing and consolidating the kidneys and astringing the essence alone cannot treat this problem in its entirety. Because of this, recurrence of spermatorrhea is likely as soon as consolidating and astringing therapy is suspended. Since this problem stems from the spirit not being housed properly within the heart, the *jing* cannot return to its source. Thus, rendering treatment to the heart is a crucial point in treating this problem. In this case, the qi needs to be nourished and the *shen* must be calmed. In addition, appropriate medicinals should be used to descend fire and clear the heart, as well as nourish the blood. If the spirit is to be calm within the heart, imperial fire must also be calm within the fire organ. This is the way to treat spermatorrhea with dreams.

2. *Tong yin tong yong*
Opening in the face of openness

Spermatorrhea is never a simple problem. Its etiology is usually a combination of different causes. Sometimes repletion is at fault. When it is, opening in the face of openness method should be used. This means that the etiological factor causing the spermatorrhea must be identified and eliminated before treatment can be successful. It is called opening in the face of openness since spermatorrhea, as a pathocondition, is a symptom of discharge. Normally in such cases, as with diarrhea and polyuria, one would think to stop the flow or discharge by astringing and consolidating. However, not all spermatorrhea is due to vacuity. Therefore, unless the causative factors are removed through a species of *xie fa* or draining therapy, the condition will persist. In clinical practice, this primarily implies using heat clearing and dampness disinhibiting medicinals to eliminate damp heat stagnation. These medicinals include Cortex Phellodendri (*Huang Bai*), Semen Coicis Lachryma-jobi (*Yi Mi*), Caulis Akebiae Mutong (*Mu Tong*), Sclerotium Poriae Cocoris (*Fu Ling*), Rhizoma Alismatis (*Ze Xie*), Rhizoma Dioscoreae Hypoglaucae (*Bi Xie*), Rhizoma Smilacis Glabrae (*Tu Fu Ling*), etc.

Should repletion spermatorrhea be due to liver qi stagnation, appropriate medicinals should be used to course the liver and regulate the qi. A typical appropriate formula for this condition is *Xiao Yao San*. If liver and heart fires are replete, an appropriate formula is *Long Dan Xie Gan Tang* plus Rhizoma Coptidis Chinensis (*Huang Lian*).

3. *Kai shui qiao, bi jing qiao*
Opening the water portal, closing the essence portal

The liver controls the coursing and discharge of the qi. It needs to be open and free flowing all the time in order to function properly. The kidneys, on the other hand, store the *jing*. They need to be closed in order to fulfill this function properly. Healthy sexual intercourse is both based on the liver's function of coursing and discharge and on the kidneys' function of storing the *jing*. If damp heat obstructs the liver channel, it may also stir up ministerial fire and disturb the palace of *jing*. This may then cause spermatorrhea. This type of spermatorrhea is not due to the kidneys' failure to consolidate the essence. It is, in fact, a product of excessive dispersion on the part of the liver.

The appropriate therapeutic principles for treating this kind of spermatorrhea are to clear heat and disinhibit dampness in the liver channel via discharging these through the water portals. Once damp heat is clear and eliminated in the liver channel and the liver is thus subdued, the palace of *jing* will be peaceful and undisturbed. Then this kind of spermatorrhea will not occur. Thus it is said, "When the water portals are opened, the essence portal is safely closed."

Bian zheng lun zhi
Treatment based on pattern discrimination

There are two main ways one can discriminate patterns in the TCM treatment of spermatorrhea. These are organ/bowel pattern discrimination (*zang fu bian zheng*) and disease cause pattern discrimination (*bing yin bian zheng*).

A. Organ/bowel pattern discrimination

1. *Shen qi bu gu*
Kidney qi not consolidating/consolidated

Pathognomic manifestations: Soreness of the lumbar region, weakness of the knees and legs, loosening of the teeth, loss of hair, impotence, seminal emission, frequent urination, nocturia, premature ejaculation, and a deep, weak pulse

Therapeutic principles: Supplement the kidneys and consolidate or secure the *jing*

Guiding formulas:

He Che Da Zao Wan

Placenta Hominis (*Zi He Che*)
Radix Panacis Ginseng (*Ren Shen*)
Radix Coquitus Rehmanniae (*Shu Di*)

Cortex Eucommiae Ulmoidis (*Du Zhong*)
Tuber Asparagi Cochinensis (*Tian Dong*)
Tuber Ophiopogonis Japonicae (*Mai Dong*)
Plastrum Testudinis (*Gui Ban*)
Cortex Phellodendri (*Huang Bai*)
Sclerotium Poriae Cocoris (*Fu Ling*)
Radix Achyranthis Bidentatae (*Huai Niu Xi*)

Jin Suo Gu Jing Wan

Fructus Rosae Laevigatae (*Jin Ying Zi*)
Herba Cynomorii Songarici (*Suo Yang*)
Semen Astragali (*Sha Yuan Ji Li*)
Semen Euryalis Ferocis (*Qian Shi*)
Semen Nelumbinis Nuciferae (*Lian Zi*)
Stamen Nelumbinis Nuciferae (*Lian Xu*)
Os Draconis (*Long Gu*)
Concha Ostreae (*Mu Li*)

2. Shen xin bu jiao
Loss of communication between the kidneys & heart

Pathognomic manifestations: Spermatorrhea with or without dreams, and accompanied by such yin vacuity symptoms as lower back and knee soreness and weakness, restlessness, palpitations, forgetfulness, dizziness, a red tongue with scant coating, and a thready, rapid pulse

Therapeutic principles: Reestablish communication of connection between the heart and kidneys

Guiding formula: San Cai Feng Sui Dan

Tuber Ophiopogonis Japonicae (*Mai Dong*), 60g
Radix Coquitus Rehmanniae (*Shu Di Huang*), 60g
Radix Panacis Ginseng (*Ren Shen*), 70g
Cortex Phellodendri (*Huang Bai*), 90g

Fructus Seu Semen Amomi (*Sha Ren*), 15g
Radix Praeparatus Glycyrrhizae (*Zhi Gan Cao*), 20g

Make into pills.

3. *Shen yin xu*
Kidney yin vacuity

Pathognomic manifestations: Feverish sensations in the palms and soles, insomnia with mental restlessness, malar flushing, dry mouth at night, tidal fever, night sweats, soreness of he lumbar region, weakness of the knees and legs, tinnitus or deafness, seminal emission, a red tongue with scant coating, and a deep, thready, rapid pulse

Therapeutic principles: Supplement the kidneys and enrich yin

Guiding formulas:

Zhi Bai Di Huang Wan

Cortex Phellodendri (*Huang Bai*)
Rhizoma Anemarrhenae (*Zhi Mu*)
Radix Coquitus Rehmanniae (*Shu Di*)
Fructus Corni Officinalis (*Shan Zhu Yu*)
Radix Dioscoreae Oppositae (*Shan Yao*)
Sclerotium Poriae Cocoris (*Fu Ling*)
Cortex Radicis Moutan (*Dan Di*)
Rhizoma Alismatis (*Ze Xie*)

Da Bu Yin Wan

Rhizoma Anemarrhenae (*Zhi Mu*)
Cortex Phellodendri (*Huang Bai*)
Radix Coquitus Rehmanniae (*Shu Di*)
Plastrum Testudinis (*Gui Ban*)
Pig bone marrow (*Zhu Ji Sui*)

4. *Gan huo wang*
Liver fire effulgence

Pathognomic manifestations: Red, swollen eyes, swelling and ulcers in the scrotal region, irascibility, headache, a bitter taste in the mouth, a red tongue with yellow coating, and a rapid, wiry pulse

Therapeutic principles: Soothe the liver and discharge fire

Guiding formulas:

Gou Zhi Qing Gan Tang

Ramulus Uncariae Cum Uncis (*Gou Teng*), 15g
Fructus Gardeniae Jasminoidis (*Zhi Zi*), 9g
Radix Gentianae Scabrae (*Long Dan Cao*), 9g
Fructus Meliae Toosendanis (*Jin Ling Zi*), 9g
Sclerotium Rubrum Poriae Cocoris (*Chi Fu Ling*), 9g
Radix Angelicae Sinensis (*Dang Gui*), 9g
Cortex Radicis Moutan (*Dan Pi*), 9g
Radix Bupleuri (*Chai Hu*), 6g
Radix Glycyrrhizae (*Gan Cao*), 3g

Long Dan Xie Gan Tang

Radix Gentianae Scabrae (*Long Dan Cao*)
Radix Scutellariae Baicalensis (*Huang Qin*)
Fructus Gardeniae Jasminoidis (*Zhi Zi*)
Rhizoma Alismatis (*Ze Xie*)
Semen Plantaginis (*Che Qian Zi*)
Caulis Akebiae Mutong (*Mu Tong*)
Radix Rehmanniae (*Sheng Di*)
Apex Radicis Angelicae Sinensis (*Dang Gui Wei*)
Radix Bupleuri (*Chai Hu*)
Radix Glycyrrhizae (*Gan Cao*)

5. *Xin huo bu an*
Heart fire not calm

Pathognomic manifestations: Palpitations, vexatious heat in the chest, ulceration, swelling, and pain of the mouth and tongue, frequency and urgency of urination, a red tongue

Therapeutic principles: Clear heart fire and calm the *shen*

Guiding formula: *Qing Xin Tang Jia Huang Lian*

Radix Rehmanniae (*Sheng Di*)
Radix Salviae Miltiorrhizae (*Dan Shen*)
Concha Ostreae (*Mu Li*)
Fructus Rosae Laevigatae (*Jin Ying Zi*)
Radix Dioscoreae Oppositae (*Shan Yao*)
Cortex Phellodendri (*Huang Bai*)
Semen Plantaginis (*Che Qian Zi*)
Fructus Schizandrae Chinensis (*Wu Wei Zi*)
Radix Polygalae Tenuifloiae (*Yuan Zhi*)
Fructus Zizyphi Jujubae (*Da Zao*)
Sclerotium Pararadicis Poriae Cocoris (*Fu Shen*)
Tuber Ophiopogonis Japonicae (*Mai Dong*)
Rhizoma Coptidis Chinensis (*Huang Lian*)

6. *Xin pi liang kui*
Heart/spleen dual deficiency

Pathognomic manifestations: Premature ejaculation with shortness of breath, palpitations, dizziness, fatigue, poor appetite, a pale tongue, and a weak pulse

Therapeutic principles: Supplement the heart and strengthen the spleen

Guiding formulas:

Gui Pi Tang

Radix Panacis Ginseng (*Ren Shen*)
Radix Astragali Seu Hedysari (*Huang Qi*)
Radix Angelicae Sinensis (*Dang Gui*)
Arillus Euphoriae Longanae (*Long Yan Rou*)
Rhizoma Atractylodis Macrocephalae (*Bai Zhu*)
Radix Saussureae Seu Vladimiriae (*Mu Xiang*)
Sclerotium Poriae Cocoris (*Fu Ling*)
Radix Polygalae Tenuifoliae (*Yuan Zhi*)
Semen Zizyphi Spinosae (*Zao Ren*)
Radix Praeparatus Glycyrrhizae (*Zhi Gan Cao*)
Rhizoma Recens Zingiberis (*Sheng Jiang*)
Fructus Zizyphi Jujubae (*Da Zao*)

Ren Shen Yang Rong Tang

Radix Angelicae Sinensis (*Dang Gui*)
Radix Albus Paeoniae Lactiflorae (*Bai Shao*)
Radix Panacis Ginseng (*Ren Shen*)
Rhizoma Atractylodis Macrocephalae (*Bai Zhu*)
Sclerotium Poriae Cocoris (*Fu Ling*)
Radix Praeparatus Glycyrrhizae (*Zhi Gan Cao*)
Fructus Schizandrae Chinensis (*Wu Wei Zi*)
Radix Polygalae Tenuifoliae (*Yuan Zhi*)
Pericarpium Citri Reticulatae (*Chen Pi*)
Radix Astragali Seu Hedysari (*Huang Qi*)
Cortex Cinnamomi (*Rou Gui*)
Rhizoma Recens Zingiberis (*Sheng Jiang*)
Fructus Zizyphi Jujubae (*Da Zao*)

B. Disease cause pattern discrimination

1. *Xiang huo wang dong*
Reckless movement of ministerial fire

Pathognomic manifestations: Spermatorrhea with dizziness, palpitations, tinnitus, deafness, low back and knee soreness and weakness, a red tongue, and a thready pulse

Therapeutic principles: Enrich yin and descend fire

Guiding formulas:

Zhi Bai Di Huang Wan (see above)

Shui Lu Er Xian Tang

Semen Euryalis Ferocis (*Qian Shi*)
Fructus Rosae Laevigatae (*Jin Ying Zi*)

2. *Shi re xia zhu*
   Damp heat pours downward

Pathognomic manifestations: Spermatorrhea accompanied by flank pain, a bitter taste in the mouth, red eyes, turbid, dribbling urination, and a red tongue with a yellow, slimy coating

Therapeutic principles: Clear heat and disinhibit dampness

Guiding formulas:

For damp heat in the lower burner:

Rhizoma Dioscoreae Hypoglaucae (*Bi Xie*)
Cortex Phellodendri (*Huang Bai*)
Semen Plantaginis (*Che Qian Zi*)
Rhizoma Acori Graminei (*Shi Chang Pu*)
Sclerotium Poriae Cocoris (*Fu Ling*)
Herba Cum Radice Taraxaci Mongolici (*Pu Gong Ying*)
Herba Polygoni Avicularis (*Bian Xu*)
Radix Gentianae Scabrae (*Long Dan Cao*)
Talcum (*Ha Shi*)
Semen Coicis Lachryma-jobi (*Yi Yi Ren*)
Radix Glycyrrhizae (*Gan Cao*)

For damp heat in the spleen/stomach:

Bi Bai Cang Zhu Jian

Rhizoma Dioscoreae Hypoglaucae (*Bi Xie*)
Sclerotium Poriae Cocoris (*Fu Ling*)
Rhizoma Atractylodis (*Cang Zhu*)
Rhizoma Atractylodis Macrocephalae (*Bai Zhu*)
Herba Eupatorii Fortunei (*Pei Lan*)
Cortex Phellodendri (*Huang Bai*)
Radix Sophorae Flavescentis (*Ku Shen*)
Medulla Tetrapanacis Papyriferi (*Tong Cao*)
Radix Glycyrrhizae (*Gan Cao*)

3. Qi zhi xue yu
Qi stagnation, blood stasis

Pathognomic manifestations: Frequent spermatorrhea with weakness and soreness in the lumbar region, impotence, dark, lusterless facial complexion, semen outflows with urination, and a dark colored tongue

Therapeutic principles: Course the liver and regulate the qi, activate the blood and transform stasis

Guiding formula: Xue Fu Zhu Yu Tang

Semen Pruni Persicae (*Tao Ren*)
Flos Carthami Tinctorii (*Hong Hua*)
Radix Angelicae Sinensis (*Dang Gui*)
Rhizoma Ligustici Wallichii (*Chuan Xiong*)
Radix Rubrus Paeoniae Lactiflorae (*Chi Shao*)
Radix Cyathulae (*Chuan Niu Xi*)
Radix Bupleuri (*Chai Hu*)
Radix Platycodi Grandiflori (*Jie Geng*)
Fructus Citri Seu Ponciri (*Zhi Ke*)
Radix Rehmanniae (*Sheng Di*)
Radix Glycyrrhizae (*Gan Cao*)

Acupuncture/moxibustion therapy

Kidney qi not consolidating/consolidated

Drain the *Ba Liao* points and then supplement *Zhong Ji* (CV 3), *Guan Yuan* (CV 4), *Ming Men* (GV 4), and *Shen Shu* (Bl 23).

Kidney vacuity & liver depression

Use even supplementation and drainage at *Qi Men* (Liv 14) and *San Yin Jiao* (Sp 6).

Kidney/spleen dual vacuity

Supplement *Zu San Li* (St 36), *Zhong Wan* (CV 12), and *San Yin Jiao* (Sp 6).

Loss of communication between the heart & kidneys

Use even supplementation and drainage at *Nei Guan* (Per 6) and *Shen Men* (Ht 7). Or, use electrostimulation at *Zhong Ji* (CV 3), *Guan Yuan* (CV 4), *Zhong Wan* (CV 12), *San Yin Jiao* (Sp 6), *Zu San Li* (ST 36), *Bai Hui* (GV 20), *Yin Tang* (M-HN-3), and *Shen Men* (Ht 7).

Zao xie
Premature ejaculation

There are several different classifications of premature ejaculation: ejaculation prior to intromission, ejaculation at the time of initial penetration, and involuntary ejaculation before the woman achieves orgasm. This is a common male sexual dysfunction. Often, problems with premature ejaculation are associated with impotence and spermatorrhea. In fact, these three problems can form a progression with problems with premature ejaculation manifesting first, followed or accompanied by spermatorrhea, and culminating in eventual impotence. Therefore, TCM practitioners think that it is important to treat premature ejaculation beyond its being extremely psychologically upsetting to the patient.

Bing yin bing ji
Disease causes, disease mechanisms

Premature ejaculation, like spermatorrhea, belongs to the *jing bing* or essence diseases. Its cause is primarily the loss of communication and connection between the heart and kidneys. This is mostly due to emotional upset and overtaxation. Water and fire thus fail to interact properly and fail to keep closed the essence portal. however, in some cases, premature ejaculation can be due to kidney yang not consolidating. This is mostly encountered in older men and is due to aging.

Bian zheng lun zhi
Treatment based on pattern discrimination

1. *Xin shen bu jiao*
Loss of communication between the heart & kidneys

Pathognomic manifestations: Premature ejaculation, vexatious heat in the five centers, dizziness, tinnitus, night sweats, lack of strength, soreness and weakness of the low back and knees, a red tongue with a thin, yellow coating, and a thready, rapid pulse

Therapeutic principles: Enrich yin and descend fire, astringe the *jing* and stop discharge

Guiding formulas: *Zhi Bai Di Huang Wan* plus ***Jin Suo Gu Jing Wan*** (see above)

In the treatment of premature ejaculation, caution must be taken not to use too many bitter, cold medicinals or hot, warm medicinals. Bitter, cold medicinals can injure the kidney qi, which then may fail to secure the palace of *jing*. Hot, warm medicinals in excess may give rise to ministerial fire disturbing the palace of *jing*, thus forcing the *jing* to leak out of the body. It is also of utmost importance that the patient's psychological fears regarding premature ejaculation be addressed during therapy if success is to be achieved.

2. Yang xu bu gu
Yang vacuity not consolidating

Pathognomic manifestations: Premature ejaculation, shortness of breath, heart palpitations, spontaneous sweating, lack of strength, fear of cold and chilled extremities, chilly pain of the low back, a white face, clear, frequent urination, spirit exhausted, feeble voice, a pale tongue, and a weak pulse

Therapeutic principles: Warm the yang and consolidate the *jing*, supplement the kidneys and boost the qi

Guiding formula: Gui Fu Du Jin Zan Yu Dan

Cortex Cinnamomi (*Rou Gui*), 60g
Radix Praeparatus Aconiti Carmichaeli (*Zhi Fu Zi*) 60g
Cortex Eucommiae Ulmoidis (*Du Zhong*), 125 g
Fructus Rosae Laevigatae (*Jin Ying Zi*), 125g
Radix Coquitus Rehmanniae (*Shu Di*), 250g
Herba Epimedii (*Yin Yang Huo*), 250g
Rhizoma Atractylodis Macrocephalae (*Bai Zhu*), 250g
Fructus Lycii Chinensis (*Gou Qi*), 180g
Radix Angelicae Sinensis (*Dang Gui*), 180g
Fructus Corni Officinalis (*Shan Zhu Yu*), 125g
Semen Euryalis Ferocis (*Qian Shi*), 125g
Rhizoma Curculiginis Orchoidis (*Xian Mao*), 125g
Semen Cnidii Monnieri (*She Chuang Zi*), 125g
Semen Allii Tuberosi (*Jiu Cai Zi*), 125g
Herba Cistanchis (*Rou Cong Rong*), 125g
Radix Morindae Officinalis (*Ba Ji Tian*), 125g

Grind into powder and make into pills with honey. Each pill should weigh 6g. Take 1 pill each time, 2-3 times per day.

External treatment:

Decoct equal amounts of Semen Cnidii Monnieri (*She Chuang Zi*) and Cortex Radicis Lycii (*Di Gu Pi*) and use as a wash prior to intercourse.

Bu she jing
Failure to ejaculate

Failure to ejaculate during intercourse is another male sexual dysfunction disease covered by TCM *nan ke* or urology. It is one of the most common causes of male infertility.

Bing yin bing ji
Disease causes, disease mechanisms

The disease mechanisms causing failure to ejaculate can be divided into two basic groups: 1) evil repletion obstructing the palace of *jing* and 2) weakness of the righteous qi not allowing for opening of the palace of *jing*. Evil qi obstructing the free flow of *jing* from the palace of *jing* include liver qi, blood stasis, and phlegm dampness. These may accumulate due to injury of the seven passions or attacks of the six evils affecting the organs and bowels as well as faulty diet and lifestyle. In addition, failure to ejaculate may also be due to righteous qi vacuity and insufficiency of *jing* essence. This may be due to chronic disease, age, taxation, poor diet, or any number of factors causing vacuity and deficiency.

In particular, because the liver controls both the sinews and coursing and discharge, the free flow of liver qi is closely connected to the free and unobstructed flow of the *jing*. Therefore, injury of the seven passions affecting the liver can often set in motion a number of pathological changes resulting in obstruction of the palace of *jing*. In Chinese medicine, the penis is spoken of as the reunion of the hundred sinews. Also, *jing*, qi, and *shen* are all closely related to liver function. When these three are healthy and balanced, normal ejaculation can occur. Dispersion of liver qi assures calmness of the *shen*. Sufficiency of liver blood insures fullness of kidney *jing*. With the dispersion of the liver, the palace of *jing* is free to open and close and hence ejaculation is normal.

On the other hand, liver qi stagnation causes depression of the spirit. This in turn results in failure to ejaculate. Because the liver channel traverses the external genitalia, any disturbance in liver function can greatly impact ejaculatory function. Therefore, depression of the liver is an important cause of failure to ejaculate.

Bian zheng lun zhi
Treatment based on pattern discrimination

1. Gan yu qi zhi
Liver depression, qi stagnation

Pathognomic manifestations: Irritability, mental depression, chest oppression, sighing, dizziness, abdominal distention and pain, cold hands when nervous or under stress which warm up when relaxed, and a wiry pulse

Therapeutic principles: Course the liver and regulate the qi

Guiding formulas:

Si Ni San

Radix Bupleuri (*Chai Hu*)
Fructus Immaturus Citri Seu Ponciri (*Zhi Shi*)
Radix Albus Paeoniae Lactiflorae (*Bai Shao*)
Radix Glycyrrhizae (*Gan Cao*)

Kai Yu Zhong Yu Tang

Radix Albus Paeoniae Lactiflorae (*Bai Shao*)
Radix Angelicae Sinensis (*Dang Gui*)
Rhizoma Atractylodis Macrocephalae (*Bai Zhu*)
Sclerotium Poriae Cocoris (*Fu Ling*)
Cortex Radicis Moutan (*Dan Pi*)
Rhizoma Cyperi Rotundi (*Xiang Fu*)
Radix Trichosanthis Kirlowii (*Tian Ha Fen*)

2. Gan yu shen xu
Liver depression, kidney vacuity

Pathognomic manifestations: Chest oppression, flank pain, irritability, frequent urination, nocturia, low back soreness, soreness and weakness of the knees and leg, tinnitus, dizziness, poor memory, and a deep, possibly thready, wiry pulse

Therapeutic principles: Nourish the liver and supplement the kidneys, boost the *jing* and open the portal

Guiding formula: *Tong Jing Yi Fang*

Semen Cuscutae (*Tu Si Zi*), 20g
Lignum Cudraniae Cochinensis (*Chuan Bo Shi*), 20g
Fructus Liquidambaris Taiwanianae (*Lu Lu Tong*), 20g
Fructus Lycii Chinensis (*Gou Qi Zi*), 15g
Fructus Ligustri Lucidi (*Nu Zhen Zi*), 15g
Herba Ecliptae Prostratae (*Han Lian Cao*), 15g
Radix Salviae Miltiorrhizae (*Dan Shen*), 15g
Herba Epimedii (*Xian Ling Pi*), 12g
Tuber Curcumae (*Yu Jin*), 10g
Cortex Radicis Moutan (*Dan Pi*), 10g

3. Gan dan shi re
Liver/gallbladder damp heat

Pathognomic manifestations: Failure to ejaculate, with red eyes, a bitter taste in the mouth, restlessness, abdominal pain and distention, a red tongue with yellow coating, and a rapid, wiry pulse

Therapeutic principles: Clear heat and disinhibit dampness

Guiding formula: *Long Dan Xie Gan Tang* (see above)

4. Gan yu pi xu
Liver depression, spleen vacuity

Pathognomic manifestations: Failure to ejaculate, chest pain, poor digestion, a bitter taste in the mouth, sluggishness of the whole body, a pale tongue, and a wiry pulse

Therapeutic principles: Drain the liver and strengthen the spleen

Guiding formula: *Xiao Yao San* plus *Gui Pi Tang*

Xiao Yao San (see above)

Gui Pi Tang

Radix Panacis Ginseng (*Ren Shen*)
Radix Astragali Seu Hedysari (*Huang Qi*)
Radix Angelicae Sinensis (*Dang Gui*)
Arillus Euphoriae Longanae (*Long Yan Rou*)
Rhizoma Atractylodis Macrocephalae (*Bai Zhu*)
Radix Saussureae Seu Vladimiriae (*Mu Xiang*)
Sclerotium Poriae Cocoris (*Fu Ling*)
Radix Polygalae Tenuifoliae (*Yuan Zhi*)
Semen Zizyphi Spinosae (*Suan Zao Ren*)
Radix Praeparatus Glycyrrhizae (*Zhi Gan Cao*)
Rhizoma Recens Zingiberis (*Sheng Jiang*)
Fructus Zizyphi Jujubae (*Da Zao*)

5. *Shen pi liang xu jia shi zu*
   Kidney/spleen dual vacuity with accumulation of dampness

Pathognomic manifestations: Failure to ejaculate, low back and knee soreness and pain, poor digestion, tinnitus, insomnia, a pale tongue, and a deep, slippery pulse

Therapeutic principles: Nourish the kidneys and strengthen the spleen, transform dampness and disinhibit the portal

Guiding formula: *Tong Jing Er Fang*

Semen Cuscutae (*Tu Si Zi*), 20g
Lignum Cudraniae Cochinensis (*Chuan Bo Shi*), 20g

Radix Codonopsis Pilosulae (*Dang Shen*), 20g
Fructus Liquidambaris Taiwanianae (*Lu Lu Tong*), 20g
Sclerotium Poriae Cocoris (*Fu Ling*), 20g
Herba Epimedii (*Yin Yang Huo*), 12g
Herba Cynomorii Songarici (*Suo Yang*), 15g
Rhizoma Atractylodis Macrocephalae (*Bai Zhu*), 10g
Pericarpium Viridis Citri Reticulatae (*Qing Pi*), 10g
Semen Pruni Armeniacae (*Xing Ren*), 10g
Rhizoma Acori Graminei (*Shi Chang Pu*), 6g
Semen Coicis Lachryma-jobi (*Yi Yi Ren*), 18g

6. *Shen yin xu*
Kidney yin vacuity

Pathognomic manifestations: Failure to ejaculate, nocturia, dry mouth and throat, low back and knee soreness and pain, dizziness, a red tongue with scant or no coating, and a thready, rapid pulse

Therapeutic principles: Enrich the kidneys and nourish yin

Guiding formulas:

Da Bu Yin Wan (see above)

Liu Wei Di Huang Wan

Radix Coquitus Rehmanniae (*Shu Di*)
Fructus Corni Officinalis (*Shan Zhu Yu*)
Radix Dioscoreae Oppositae (*Shan Yao*)
Sclerotium Poriae Cocoris (*Fu Ling*)
Cortex Radicis Moutan (*Dan Pi*)
Rhizoma Alismatis (*Ze Xie*)

7. *Shen yin xu, xiang huo wang dong*
Kidney yin vacuity, reckless stirring of ministerial fire

Pathognomic manifestations: Failure to ejaculate, polyuria, nocturia, tinnitus, red eyes, mouth sores, dream disturbed sleep, restlessness, insomnia, a red tongue, and a thready, rapid pulse

Therapeutic principles: Nourish yin and descend fire

Guiding formula: *Zhi Bai Di Huang Wan* (see above)

8. *Shen xu jing qiao bi*
Kidney vacuity, *jing* portal closed shut

Pathognomic manifestations: Failure to ejaculate plus polyuria, nocturia, tinnitus, dizziness, low back and knee soreness and weakness, cold lower extremities, chronic fatigue, poor memory, a pale tongue with thin, white coating, and a deep, weak, possibly slow pulse

Therapeutic principles: Supplement the kidneys and open the *jing* portal

Guiding formula: *Bu Shen Yi Qi Tong Jing Tang*

Radix Coquitus Rehmanniae (*Shu Di*) 25g
Radix Dioscoreae Oppositae (*Shan Yao*), 15g
Radix Codonopsis Pilosulae (*Dang Shen*), 15g
Radix Astragali Seu Hedysari (*Huang Qi*), 20g
Radix Salviae Miltiorrhizae (*Dan Shen*), 20g
Semen Astragali (*Sha Yuan Zi*), 12g
Semen Cuscutae (*Tu Si Zi*), 12g
Radix Angelicae Sinensis (*Dang Gui*), 12g
Fructus Liquidambaris Taiwanianae (*Lu Lu Tong*), 12g
Semen Cnidii Monnieri (*She Chuan Zi*), 10g
Herba Epimedii (*Xian Ling Pi*), 10g
Ramulus Cinnamomi (*Gui Zhi*), 10g

9. *Qi zhi xue yu*
Qi stagnation, blood stasis

Pathognomic manifestations: Failure to ejaculate, chest pain, insomnia, easily angered, purple petechiae on the tongue, and a wiry and/or grating/astringent pulse

Therapeutic principles: Activate the blood and transform stasis, move the qi and open the portal

Guiding formula: *Xue Fu Zhu Yu Tang* (see above)

10. *Tan zhuo jing bi*
Phlegm turbidity obstructing the *jing*

Pathognomic manifestations: Failure to ejaculate, spermator-rhea, forgetfulness, irritability, short, yellow urine, a dark, purplish tongue with slimy coating, and a slippery, rapid, forceful pulse

Therapeutic principles: Eliminate dampness, transform phlegm, and open the portals

Guiding formulas:

Bi Xie Fen Qing Yin

Rhizoma Dioscoreae Hypoglaucae (*Bi Xie*)
Fructus Alpiniae Oxyphyllae (*Yi Zhi Ren*)
Radix Linderae Strychnifoliae (*Wu Yao*)
Rhizoma Acori Graminei (*Shi Chang Pu*)

Er Chen Tang

Rhizoma Pinelliae Ternatae (*Ban Xia*)
Pericarpium Citri Reticulatae (*Chen Pi*)
Sclerotium Poriae Cocoris (*Fu Ling*)
Radix Glycyrrhizae (*Gan Cao*)

Acupuncture/moxibustion therapy

Liver depression, kidney vacuity:

Drain *Zhong Ji* (CV 3) and *Xing Jian* (Liv 2). Supplement *San Yin Jiao* (Sp 6) and *Shen Shu* (Bl 23).

Liver depression, spleen vacuity:

Drain *Da Dun* (Liv 1) and moxa *Zu San Li* (St 36). Needle *Qu Gu* (CV 2) and *Yin Lian* (Liv 11).

Electrical stimulation

Guan Yuan (CV 4), *Zhong Ji* (CV 3), *Qu Gu* (CV 2), *Ba Liao* (Bl 31-34), *Hui Yin* (CV 1), and *Shen Shu* (Bl 23)

Xue jing
Bloody semen

Xue jing means bloody semen or blood in the semen, and is another common male urological condition. It is encountered in such modern Western diseases as prostatitis, vesiculitis, prostate cancer, etc.

Bing yin bing ji
Disease causes, disease mechanisms

Blood in the semen is a bleeding disorder. Therefore, its causes and mechanisms are similar to other bleeding disorders. There are four mechanisms involved with abnormal bleeding. These are heat, qi vacuity, stasis, and trauma. In terms of bloody semen, the first three are the most commonly met mechanisms.

Most often, bloody semen is due to heat causing the blood to run recklessly outside its pathways. This heat can be either replete or vacuous. If the heat is replete, it is most often damp heat. Damp heat may accumulate in the palace of *jing*, damaging the vessels and thus causing the blood to leak out. Such dampness and heat may be due to a combination of depressive liver heat due to emotional causes, with spleen dysfunction due to faulty diet. It may also be due to overeating greasy, spicy foods. Vacuity heat is mostly due to aging, chronic disease, overtaxation, excessive sex, drug abuse, and other such factors.

Qi vacuity may result in the qi's failure to restrain the blood within its vessels. This is most commonly due to spleen vacuity, in turn due to overtaxation or faulty diet. However, it may also be due to kidney qi vacuity failing to astringe the yin portals.

Blood stasis results in bleeding if this stasis forces the blood outside its pathways. Blood stasis may be due to trauma, including the iatrogenic sequelae of vasectomy, prolonged qi stagnation failing to move the blood, prolonged dampness and heat obstructing the free flow of the blood, or cold congealing the blood. Therefore, in clinical practice, one must distinguish between hot blood stasis and cold. It is also common for blood stasis to complicate other patterns of bloody semen, in which case appropriate blood-activating, stasis-transforming or dispelling ingredients should be added to the guiding prescriptions suggested below.

Bian zheng lun zhi
Treatment based on pattern discrimination

1. Xu re
Vacuity heat

Pathognomic manifestations: Bloody semen, irritability, restlessness, dry mouth, dry throat, red eyes, itching skin (especially on the genitalia), painful intercourse, a red tongue with scant coating, and a thready, rapid pulse

Therapeutic principles: Nourish yin, clear heat, cool the blood, and stop bleeding

Guiding formula:

Rhizoma Anemarrhenae (*Zhi Mu*), 20g
Cortex Phellodendri (*Huang Bai*), 20g
Rhizoma Smilacis Glabrae (*Tu Fu Ling*), 20g
Fructus Ligustri Lucidi (*Nu Zhen Zi*), 15g
Cortex Radicis Moutan (*Dan Pi*), 10g
Herba Cirsii Japonici (*Da Ji*), 10g
Herba Cephalanopoloris Segeti (*Xiao Ji*), 10g

Radix Carbonisatus Sanguisorbae (*Di Yu Tan*), 10g
Semen Plantaginis (*Che Qian Zi*), 10g
Plumula Nelumbinis Nuciferae (*Lian Zi Xin*), 10g
Radix Pseudostellariae Heterophyllae (*Tai Zi Shen*), 10g
Radix Astragali Seu Hedysari (*Huang Qi*), 10g
Fructus Meliae Toosendanis (*Chuan Lian Zi*), 10g

2. *Shi re*
Damp heat

Pathognomic manifestations: Red-colored seminal fluid, distention and pain in the penis or testicles, frequent, astringent, yellow urination, a red face and eyes, dizziness, vexation and agitation, a bitter taste in the mouth and dry throat, dry stools, a slimy, yellow tongue coating, and a slippery, wiry, rapid pulse if the condition is one of merely repletion, or a sodden rapid pulse if there is concomitant spleen qi vacuity

Therapeutic principles: Clear heat, disinhibit dampness, cool the blood, and stop bleeding

Guiding formula: *Long Dan Xie Gan Tang Jia Jian*

Radix Bupleuri (*Chai Hu*), 15g
Fructus Gardeniae Jasminoidis (*Zhi Zi*), 20g
Radix Rehmanniae (*Sheng Di*), 20g
Radix Angelicae Sinensis (*Dang Gui*), 20g
Caulis Akebiae Mutong (*Mu Tong*), 20g
Radix Scutellariae Baicalensis (*Huang Qin*), 10g
Cortex Radicis Moutan (*Dan Pi*), 10g
Radix Rubrus Paeoniae Lactiflorae (*Chi Shao*), 10g
Semen Plantaginis (*Che Qian Zi*), 25g
Radix Gentianae Scabrae (*Long Dan Cao*), 25g
Talcum (*Ha Shi*), 25g

In chronic cases, one must also add ingredients to boost the qi and consolidate the *jing* in addition to the above methods of clearing heat and disinhibiting dampness. If kidney qi is not consolidating the essence, add *Jin Gui Shen Qi Wan* a.k.a. *Ba Wei Di Huang Wan*. If spleen qi is vacuous, add *Bu Zhong Yi Qi Tang*.

3. *Pi qi xu*
Spleen qi vacuity

Pathognomic manifestations: Reddish seminal fluid, a heavy sensation in the entire body, lack of appetite, poor digestion, a pale face, a pale tongue with thin, white coating, and a deep, weak pulse

Therapeutic principles: Supplement the spleen and boost the qi

Guiding formula: *Bu Zhong Yi Qi Tang* (see above)

4. *Shen qi bu bu*
Kidney qi not consolidating/consolidated

Pathognomic manifestations: Red colored seminal fluid, dizziness and tinnitus, spiritual exhaustion and lack of strength, loss of sleep with many dreams, soreness and weakness of the low back and knees, a red tongue with a thin, white coating, and thready, forceless pulse

Therapeutic principles: Consolidate and nourish kidney *jing*, strengthen the spleen and boost the qi

Guiding formula:

Shen Qi Wan a.k.a. ***Ba Wei Di Huang Wan*** (see above)

Liu Wei Di Huang Wan He Bu Zhong Yi Qi Tang Jia Jian

Radix Coquitus Rehmanniae (*Shu Di*)
Fructus Corni Officinalis (*Shan Zhu Yu*)
Radix Dioscoreae Oppositae (*Shan Yao*)
Rhizoma Alismatis (*Ze Xie*)
Cortex Radicis Moutan (*Dan Pi*)
Sclerotium Poriae Cocoris (*Fu Ling*)

Radix Codonopsis Pilosulae (*Dang Shen*)
Radix Astragali Seu Hedysari (*Huang Qi*)
Radix Angelicae Sinensis (*Dang Gui*)
Gelatinum Corii Asini (*E Jiao*)
Pollen Typhae (*Sheng Pu Huang*)
Cortex Eucommiae Ulmoidis (*Du Zhong*)
Cacumen Carbonisatus Biotae (*Ce Bai Tan*)
Radix Praeparatus Glycyrrhizae (*Zhi Gan Cao*)

5. *Xue yu*
Blood stasis

A. *Re xing*
Hot pattern

Pathognomic manifestations: Reddish seminal fluid, a painful sensation in the testicles, painful intercourse, a red face, restlessness, irritability, constipation, a red tongue with yellow coating, and a rapid pulse

Therapeutic principles: Clear heat and discharge the bowels, activate the blood and dispel stasis

Guiding formulas:

Tao He Cheng Qi Tang (see above)

One may add medicinals to resolve toxins, cool the blood, and stop bleeding as appropriate, such as Radix Salviae Miltiorrhizae (*Dan Shen*), Pollen Typhae (*Sheng Pu Huang*), Rhizoma Imperatae Cylindricae (*Bai Mao Geng*), Cacumen Carbonisatus Biotae (*Ce Bai Tan*), Radix Rehmanniae (*Sheng Di*), Herba Cirsii Japonicae (*Da Ji*), and Herba Cephalanopoloris Segeti (*Xiao Ji*).

Unnamed formula

Herba Agrimoniae Pilosae (*Xian He Cao*), 15g
Herba Ecliptae Prostratae (*Han Lian Cao*), 15g
Fructus Zizyphi Jujubae (*Da Zao*), 15 pieces

Unnamed formula

Nodus Rhizomatis Nelumbinis Nuciferae (*Ou Jie*), 20g
Crinis Carbonisatus (*Xue Yu Tan*)

These last two formulas treat bloody semen with pain and frequent urination.

B. *Han xing*
   Cold pattern

Pathognomic manifestations: Bloody semen, cold abdomen and testicles, cold limbs, a pale face, and a slow pulse

Therapeutic principles: Dispel cold, transform stasis, and stop bleeding

Guiding formula: *Shao Fu Zhu Yu Tang* (see above)

Jing ye yi chang
Anomalies in the semen

Jing shao
Low sperm count

Low sperm count, also known as spermacrasia or oligospermia, refers to an abnormally reduced number of sperm in the ejaculate. A low sperm count can contribute to troubles conceiving. Modern Western medicine says that this condition may be idiopathic or may be associated with decreased spermatogenesis as seen with a varicocele. A sperm density of less than 200 million per milliliter makes fertilization statistically less likely.

Bing yin bing ji
Disease causes, disease mechanisms

If idiopathic, TCM mostly ascribes this condition to insufficiency of kidney yin or kidney yang vacuity resulting in vacuity and coldness of the *jing*. Kidney yin vacuity may be due to congenital insufficiency, aging, chronic disease, or chronic taxation, including physical, emotional, and sexual taxation, drug use, etc. In this case, there is insufficient yin substance to provide the material basis for spermatogenesis. In the case of kidney yang vacuity, insufficient yang qi fails to catalyze the creation and transformation of the *jing*, while cold can retard the *jing*'s free flow. Kidney yang vacuity may also be due to congenital insufficiency, aging, chronic disease, taxation, and drug use. Whether a person suffers from yang vacuity or yin vacuity is often a matter of constitutional predisposition.

However, not all cases of lowered sperm count are due to deficiency and vacuity. Oligospermia may also be due to evil repletion. Damp heat, generated due to faulty diet or stagnant qi transforming into depressive heat, may obstruct the free and patent flow of the *jing*. Likewise, qi stagnation due to emotional frustration and blood stasis may also impede and obstruct the flow of the *jing*, as may phlegm dampness and cold dampness. Typically, oligospermia even when due to an evil repletion is complicated by kidney vacuity. Therefore, in the formulas given below, all include kidney and *jing* essence supplementing medicinals.

Bian zheng lun zhi
Treatment based on pattern discrimination

1. Shen yang xu
Kidney yang vacuity

Pathognomic manifestations: Low sperm count, tinnitus, dizziness, low back and knee soreness and weakness, cold lower extremities, polyuria, nocturia, a pale tongue with thin, white coating, and a deep, slow pulse

Therapeutic principles: Supplement the kidneys and warm the *jing*

Guiding formula: *Shi Zi Wan*

To the ingredients of *Wu Zi Heng Zhong Wan* discussed above, add:

Fructus Mori Albi (*Sang Shen Zi*)
Radix Praeparatus Aconiti Carmichaeli (*Pao Fu Zi*)
Semen Allii Tuberosi (*Jiu Cai Zi*)
Semen Trigonellae Foeni-greaci (*Lu Ba Zi*)
Semen Cnidii Monnieri (*She Chuang Zi*)
Radix Angelicae Sinensis (*Dang Gui*)
Radix Dipsaci (*Chuang Xu Duan*)
Radix Codonopsis Pilosulae (*Dang Shen*)
Radix Morindae Officinalis (*Ba Ji Tian*)
Colla Cornu Cervi (*Lu Jiao Jiao*)

2. *Shen yang xu*
Kidney yin vacuity

Pathognomic manifestations: Low sperm count, low back soreness and weakness, polyuria, nocturia, restlessness, insomnia, poor memory, malar flushing in the afternoon and early evenings, tinnitus, dizziness, a red tongue with scant coating, and a thready, rapid pulse

Therapeutic principles: Supplement the kidneys, nourish yin, and generate *jing*

Guiding formula: *Ye Ha Sheng Jing Tang*

Cortex Radicis Moutan (*Dan Pi*)
Cortex Radicis Lycii (*Di Gu Pi*)
Radix Rubrus Paeoniae Lactiflorae (*Chi Shao*)
Radix Albus Paeoniae Lactiflorae (*Bai Shao*)
Fructus Corni Officinalis (*Shan Yu Rou*)
Fructus Forsythiae Suspensae (*Lian Qiao*)

Spica Prunellae Vulgaris (*Xia Gu Cao*)
Radix Bupleuri (*Chai Hu*)
Herba Lophatheri Gracilis (*Zhu Ye*)
Sclerotium Poriae Cocoris (*Fu Ling*)
Radix Rehmanniae (*Sheng Di*)
Radix Scrophulariae Ningpoensis (*Xuan Shen*)
Tuber Ophiopogonis Japonicae (*Mai Dong*)
Bulbus Fritillariae Thunbergii (*Zhe Bei Mu*)
Radix Salviae Miltiorrhizae (*Dan Shen*)
Fructus Lycii Chinensis (*Gou Qi Zi*)
Herba Epimedii (*Xian Ling Pi*)
Concha Ostreae (*Sheng Mu Li*)

3. *Pi shen liang kui*
Spleen/ kidneys both deficient

Pathognomic manifestations: Low sperm count, poor motility, low back soreness, spermatorrhea, a pale tongue with thin, white coating, and a thready, weak pulse

Therapeutic principles: Supplement the kidneys and strengthen the spleen, boost the qi and generate the *jing*

Guiding formula: *Sheng Jing Tang*

Fructus Lycii Chinensis (*Gou Qi Zi*), 15g
Radix Codonopsis Pilosulae (*Dang Shen*), 15g
Radix Dipsaci (*Chuan Xu Duan*), 15g
Radix Polygoni Multiflori (*He Shou Wu*), 15g
Semen Cuscutae (*Tu Si Zi*), 9g
Fructus Rubi (*Fu Pen Zi*), 9g
Fructus Schizandrae Chinensis (*Wu Wei Zi*), 9g
Fructus Mori Albi (*Sang Shen*), 9g
Pericarpium Citri Reticulatae (*Chen Pi*), 9g
Semen Plantaginis (*Che Qian Zi*), 9g
Radix Angelicae Sinensis (*Dang Gui*), 12g
Radix Coquitus Rehmanniae (*Shu Di*), 12g
Herba Epimedii (*Xian Ling Pi*), 12g
Radix Astragali Seu Hedysari (*Huang Qi*), 18g

4. *Gan yu shen xu*
Liver depression, kidney vacuity

Pathognomic manifestations: Low sperm count, spermatorrhea, bodily fatigue and emaciation, dizziness, tinnitus, poor sleep, excessive dreams, heart vexation, easily angered, low back and knee soreness and weakness, a red tongue with a thin, yellow coating, and a thready, rapid, and wiry pulse

Therapeutic principles: Supplement the kidneys and astringe the *jing*, clear and discharge ministerial fire

Guiding formula: *Zhi Bai Di Huang Wan Jia Jian*

Radix Coquitus Rehmanniae (*Shu Di*), 18g
Fructus Lycii Chinensis (*Gou Qi*), 8g
Semen Cuscutae (*Tu Si Zi*), 15g
Fructus Corni Officinalis (*Shan Yu Rou*), 12g
Colla Cornu Cervi (*Lu Jiao Jiao*), 12g
Radix Dioscoreae Oppositae (*Huai Shan Yao*), 12g
Sclerotium Poriae Cocoris (*Fu Ling*), 12g
Cortex Phellodendri (*Huang Bai*), 9g
Rhizoma Anemarrhenae (*Zhi Mu*), 9g
Semen Zizyphi Spinosae (*Zao Ren*), 9g
Radix Bupleuri (*Chai Hu*), 6g
Radix Achyranthis Bidentatae (*Huai Niu Xi*), 9g

5. *Tan shi zu luo*
Phlegm dampness obstructs the connecting vessels

Pathognomic manifestations: Obese body, spiritual fatigue and exhaustion, sore low back and distended abdomen, four limbs sunken and heavy, a heavy sensation in the head which is worse on cloudy days, a normal tongue or a fat tongue with teeth indentations and pale color with a white, slimy coating, and deep, thready, slippery pulse

Therapeutic principles: Transform phlegm and eliminate dampness, supplement the kidneys and boost the *jing*, open the *luo*

Guiding formula: *Fang Ji Huang Qi Tang Jia Wei*

Radix Astragali Seu Hedysari (*Huang Qi*)
Radix Stephaniae Tetrandrae (*Han Fang Ji*)
Rhizoma Atractylodis Macrocephalae (*Bai Zhu*)
Radix Praeparatus Glycyrrhizae (*Zhi Gan Cao*)
Rhizoma Recens Zingiberis (*Sheng Jiang*)
Fructus Zizyphi Jujubae (*Da Zao*)
Radix Salviae Miltiorrhizae (*Dan Shen*)
Herba Artemesiae Capillaris (*Yin Chen*)
Rhizoma Alismatis (*Ze Xie*)
Sclerotium Poriae Cocoris (*Fu Ling*)
Herba Epimedii (*Xian Ling Pi*)
Fructus Lycii Chinensis (*Gou Qi*)
Radix Polygoni Multiflori (*Shou Wu*)

6. *Xia jiao han shi*
   Cold & damp in the lower burner

Pathognomic manifestations: Low sperm count, poor motility, low back and lower abdominal soreness and pain, a heavy feeling which is worse on cloudy days, turbid urination, a feeling of astringency and pain while urinating, a slightly swollen tongue with white, greasy coating, and a surging, deep, retarded pulse which is thready and weak at both *chi* or foot positions

Therapeutic principles: Warm and transform cold and dampness

Guiding formula: *Shao Fu Zhu Yu Tang He Si Ling Tang Jia Jian*

Fructus Foeniculi Vulgaris (*Xiao Hui Xiang*), 6g
Rhizoma Praeparata Zingiberis (*Pao Jiang*), 10g
Arillus Euphoriae Longanae (*Long Yan Rou*), 10g
Radix Angelicae Sinensis (*Dang Gui*), 10g
Cortex Cinnamomi (*Rou Gui*), 6g
Radix Rubrus Paeoniae Lactiflorae (*Chi Shao*), 10g
Radix Albus Paeoniae Lactiflorae (*Bai Shao*), 13g
Rhizoma Alismatis (*Ze Xie*), 10g

Sclerotium Poriae Cocoris (*Fu Ling*), 10g
Rhizoma Dioscoreae Hypoglaucae (*Bi Xie*), 10g
Radix Achyranthis Bidentatae (*Niu Xi*), 10g

7. *Xia jiao shi re*
Damp heat in the lower burner

Pathognomic manifestations: Low sperm count, poor motility, yellow, difficult urination, painful urination, a thick yellow coating at the base of the tongue, and wiry, slippery pulse

Therapeutic principles: Clear heat and disinhibit dampness, supplement the kidneys and boost the *jing*

Guiding formulas: *Long Dan Xie Gan Tang* (see above) plus ***Liu Wei Di Huang Wan*** (see above) plus

Flos Lonicerae Japonicae (*Yin Hua*)
Fructus Forsythiae Suspensae (*Lian Qiao*)
Herba Cum Radice Taraxaci Mongolici (*Pu Gong Ying*)
Herba Violae Yedoensis (*Zi Hua Di Ding*)
Herba Patriniae Heterophyllae (*Bai Jiang Cao*)
Caulis Sargentodoxae (*Hong Teng*)
Herba Oldenlandiae Diffusae (*Bai Hua She She Cao*)

Take the *Liu Hui Di Huang Wan* in pill form and add the above herbs to the *Long Dan Xie Gan Tang* taken in decoction.

8. *Qi zhi xue yu*
Qi stagnation, blood stasis

Pathognomic manifestations: Low sperm count, poor motility, distention or discomfort in the testes or scrotum, possible purple petechiae on the tongue, and a wiry pulse

Therapeutic principles: Course the liver and regulate the qi, activate the blood and transform stasis, supplement the kidneys

Guiding formulas:

Shao Fu Zhu Yu Tang (see above)

Ge Xia Zhu Yu Tang

Radix Angelicae Sinensis (*Dang Gui*)
Rhizoma Ligustici Wallichii (*Chuan Xiong*)
Semen Pruni Persicae (*Tao Ren*)
Flos Carthami Tinctorii (*Hong Hua*)
Feces Trogopterori Seu Pteromi (*Wu Ling Zhi*)
Radix Linderae Strychnifoliae (*Wu Yao*)
Rhizoma Corydalis Yanhusuo (*Yan Hu*)
Rhizoma Cyperi Rotundi (*Xiang Fu*)
Radix Rubrus Paeoniae Lactiflorae (*Chi Shao*)
Cortex Radicis Moutan (*Dan Pi*)
Fructus Citri Seu Ponciri (*Zhi Qiao*)
Radix Glycyrrhizae (*Gan Cao*)

plus

Liu Wei Di Huang Wan (see above)

Acupuncture/moxibustion therapy

Needle *Heng Gu* (Ki 11), *Da He* (Ki 12), and *San Yin Jiao* (Sp 6).
Moxa *Zhong Ji* (CV 3), *Gui Lai* (ST 29), and *Guan Yuan* (CV 4).
Then needle the *Ba Liao* (Bl 31-34), needle and moxa *Shen Shu*
(Bl 23), and moxa *Ming Men* (GV 4).

Wu jing
Azoospermia

Azoospermia is the lack of sperm in the semen. According to
modern Western medicine, it is associated with primary testicular

disorders, complete obstruction of the seminal tract, or lack of hormonal stimulation.

Bing yin bing ji
Disease causes, disease mechanisms

The main cause of azoospermia according to TCM is kidney qi and yin vacuity. Once again, this may be due to congenital insufficiency, aging, chronic disease, or various types of taxation. In some cases, kidney vacuity is complicated by simultaneous qi stagnation and blood stasis. Qi stagnation is often due to emotional frustration and stress. Blood stasis may arise if this stagnation is prolonged or severe. Blood stasis may also be caused by trauma and the sequelae of surgery among other factors.

Bian zheng lun zhi
Treatment based on pattern discrimination

1. Qi yin liang xu
Qi & yin both vacuous

Pathognomic manifestations: Lack of sperm, poor memory, dizziness, tinnitus, gray, thinning hair, a pale face, low back soreness and weakness, a red tongue, and a deep, thready, rapid pulse

Therapeutic principles: Supplement the kidneys and boost the *jing*, consolidate the root and seal the source

Guiding formula: *Jia Jian Qi Zi San*

Fructus Schizandrae Chinensis (*Wu Wei Zi*), 10g
Semen Cuscutae (*Tu Si Zi*), 10g
Semen Plantaginis (*Che Qian Zi*), 20g
Fructus Lycii Chinensis (*Gou Qi Zi*), 15g
Herba Dendrobii (*Shi Hu*), 30g
Radix Dioscoreae Oppositae (*Tu Shan Yao*), 20g
Radix Coquitus Rehmanniae (*Shu Di Huang*), 20g

Semen Cnidii Monnieri (*She Chuang Zi*), 15g
Fructus Rosae Laevigatae (*Jin Ying Zi*), 20g
Semen Zizyphi Spinosae (*Suan Zao Ren*), 15g
Herba Cistanchis (*Rou Cong Rong*), 12g
Radix Morindae Officinalis (*Ba Ji Tian*), 6g
Sclerotium Poriae Cocoris (*Fu Ling*), 10g
Radix Panacis Quinquefolii (*Xi Yang Shen*), 15g
Radix Astragali Seu Hedysari (*Huang Qi*), 15g
Radix Praeparata Aconiti Carmichaeli (*Shu Fu Pian*), 3g
Cortex Phellodendri (*Huang Bai*), 10g

2. Shen xu jian qi zhi xue yu
Kidney vacuity with simultaneous qi stagnation & blood stasis

Pathognomic manifestations: Lack of sperm, dizziness, tinnitus, fatigue, pain and distention in the flanks, a purplish tongue, and a thready or grating/astringent pulse

Therapeutic principles: Supplement the kidneys and nourish yin, activate the blood and transform stasis

Guiding formula: Wu Zi Yan Zong Wan He Tao Hong Si Wu Tang Jia Jian

Fructus Lycii Chinensis (*Gou Qi Zi*), 20g
Semen Cuscutae (*Tu Si Zi*), 20g
Semen Plantaginis (*Che Qian Zi*), 10g
Fructus Rubi (*Fu Pen Zi*), 20g
Fructus Schizandrae Chinensis (*Wu Wei Zi*), 10g
Semen Pruni Persicae (*Tao Ren*), 3g
Flos Carthami Tinctorii (*Hong Hua*), 3g
Radix Coquitus Rehmanniae (*Shu Di*), 20g
Radix Dioscoreae Oppositae (*Shan Yao*), 20g
Fructus Corni Officinalis (*Zhu Yu*), 5g
Tuber Asparagi Cochinensis (*Tian Dong*), 20g
Tuber Ophiopogonis Japonicae (*Mai Dong*), 20g
Fructus Ligustri Lucidi (*Nu Zhen Zi*), 10g
Herba Ecliptae Prostratae (*Han Lian Cao*), 10g

Si jing
Dead sperm

Si jing or dead sperm refers to the presence of dead sperm in the ejaculate.

Bing yin bing ji
Disease causes, disease mechanisms

Based on clinical experience, modern practitioners of TCM have identified four patterns associated with dead sperm within the ejaculate. These are kidney yang emptiness, kidney yin and yang emptiness, spleen/kidney vacuity cold, and liver qi depression and stagnation.

Bian zheng lun zhi
Treatment based on pattern discrimination

1. *Shen yang xu*
Kidney yang vacuity

Pathognomic manifestations: Dead sperm within the ejaculate mostly found in older men, scant amount of seminal fluid or an excessive amount of thin, dilute semen, shortness of breath and spiritual fatigue, a pale white, lusterless face, low back ache and weak lower extremities, a chilly cold feeling in the lower abdomen, diminished sexual desire, a pale tongue with a thin coating, and a deep, weak or thready, weak pulse

Therapeutic principles: Supplement the kidneys and assist yang, warm the *jing*

Guiding formula: *Zan Yu Dan Jia Jian*

Radix Coquitus Rehmanniae (*Shu Di*), 300g

Rhizoma Atractylodis Macrocephalae (*Bai Zhu*), 300g
Radix Angelicae Sinensis (*Dang Gui*), 300g
Fructus Corni Officinalis (*Shan Zhu Yu*), 300g
Fructus Lycii Chinensis (*Gou Qi*), 300g
Radix Panacis Ginseng (*Ren Shen*), 200g
Cortex Eucommiae Ulmoidis (*Du Zhong*), 200g
Rhizoma Curculiginis Orchoidis (*Xian Mao*), 200g
Herba Epimedii (*Yin Yang Huo*), 200g
Radix Morindae Officinalis (*Ba Ji Tian*), 200g
Semen Allii Tuberosi (*Jiu Zi*), 200g
Semen Cnidii Monnieri (*She Chuang Zi*), 200g
Radix Praeparatus Aconiti Carmichaeli (*Pao Fu Zi*), 120g
Cortex Cinnamomi (*Rou Gui*), 50g
Cornu Parvum Cervi (*Lu Rong*), 100g
Secretio Moschi Moschiferi (*She Xiang*), 3g

Grind the above medicinals into a fine powder and make into pills, each pill weighing 10g. Take 1 pill each time after meals, 3 times per day.

2. *Shen yin yang ju xu*
Kidney yin & yang completely vacuous

Pathognomic manifestations: Dead sperm, spiritual fatigue, fear of chill, failure to maintain an erection during sex, a white, moist tongue coating, and a vacuous, thready, deep pulse

Therapeutic principles: Warm and supplement kidney yang, boost the qi and fill the *jing*

Guiding formula: *Zan Yu Dan Jia Jian*

Radix Coquitus Rehmanniae (*Shu Di*), 25g
Radix Praeparatus Dioscoreae Oppositae (*Chao Shan Yao*), 15g
Fructus Corni Officinalis (*Shan Yu Rou*), 15g
Radix Praeparatus Aconiti Carmichaeli (*Shu Fu Pian*), 7g
Cortex Cinnamomi (*Guang Gui*), 5g

Radix Angelicae Sinensis (*Dang Gui*), 12g
Cornu Cervi (*Lu Jiao Pian*), 30g
Radix Morindae Officinalis (*Ba Ji Rou*), 15g
Rhizoma Curculiginis Orchoidis (*Xian Mao*), 12g
Herba Epimedii (*Xian Ling Pi*), 10g
Semen Cuscutae (*Tu Si Zi*), 15g
Radix Praeparatus Astragali Seu Hedysari (*Zhi Huang Qi*), 20g
Radix Codonopsis Pilosulae (*Dang Shen*), 15g
Fructus Rosae Laevigatae (*Jin Ying Zi*), 25g
Os Draconis (*Long Gu*), 30g
Concha Ostreae (*Mu Li*), 30g

3. *Pi shen xu han*
Spleen/kidney vacuity cold

Pathognomic manifestations: Diminished seminal fluid or running, dilute fluid mostly in older men who are also sterile, diminished food intake, loss of strength, body cold, limbs chilled, shortness of breath, feeble voice, a pale tongue with a white coating, and an empty, weak pulse

Therapeutic principles: Strengthen the spleen and warm the kidneys

Guiding formula: *Bu Zhong Yi Qi Tang He Wu Zi Yan Zong Tang*

Radix Panacis Ginseng (*Ren Shen*), 15g
Radix Astragali Seu Hedysari (*Huang Qi*), 20g
Rhizoma Atractylodis Macrocephalae (*Bai Zhu*), 10g
Radix Praeparatus Glycyrrhizae (*Zhi Gan Cao*), 10g
Pericarpium Citri Reticulatae (*Chen Pi*), 10g
Fructus Schizandrae Chinensis (*Wu Wei Zi*), 10g
Cortex Cinnamomi (*Rou Gui*), 5g
Rhizoma Cimicifugae (*Sheng Ma*), 5g
Radix Bupleuri (*Chai Hu*), 5g
Radix Angelicae Sinensis (*Dang Gui*), 15g

Fructus Rubi (*Fu Pen Zi*), 20g
Semen Plantaginis (*Che Qian Zi*), 20g
Fructus Lycii Chinensis (*Gou Qi*), 20g
Semen Cuscutae (*Tu Si Zi*), 20g

4. Gan qi yu zhi
Liver qi depression & stagnation

Pathognomic manifestations: Dead sperm in the ejaculate, lower abdominal distention, weak knees, lack strength, a pale red tongue with ecchymotic spots, and a wiry, thready pulse

Therapeutic principles: Course the liver, regulate the qi, and resolve depression

Guiding formula:

Radix Bupleuri (*Chai Hu*), 9g
Radix Linderae Strychnifoliae (*Wu Yao*), 9g
Lignum Aquilariae Agallochae (*Chen Xiang*), 3g
Semen Citri (*Ju He*), 9g
Radix Albus Paeoniae Lactiflorae (*Bai Shao*), 12g
Radix Angelicae Sinensis (*Dang Gui*), 12g
Rhizoma Curculiginis Orchoidis (*Xian Mao*), 15g
Herba Epimedii (*Yin Yang Huo*), 15g
Rhizoma Cyperi Rotundi (*Xiang Fu*), 10g
Radix Glycyrrhizae (*Gan Cao*)

Jing zi huo dong lu di
Diminished sperm motility

According to modern Western medicine, diminished sperm motility is the commonest isolated abnormal seminal parameter. It may be due to varicocele or local inflammation, such as prostatitis, seminal vesiculitis, or urethritis, epididymal disease, or the presence of sperm-immobilizing or sperm-agglutinizing antibodies.

Bing yin bing ji
Disease causes, disease mechanisms

TCM primarily ascribes this sperm anomaly to kidney yang vacuity. such yang vacuity may be due to any of a number of causes. However, since yang is responsible for movement in general, it makes sense that lack of sperm motility would be due to kidney yang vacuity. Some cases are also due to both yin and yang vacuity with stirring of vacuity fire. Although vacuity fire may be responsible for the majority of the patient's signs and symptoms, still there is yang vacuity as well at the lower source.

Bian zheng lun zhi
Treatment based on pattern discrimination

1. *Shen yang bu zu*
Kidney yang insufficiency

Pathognomic manifestations: Diminished sperm motility, a pale face, dizziness, tinnitus, *jing shen* exhausted and fatigued, soreness and weakness of the low back and knees, a chilly feeling in the lower extremities, a pale tongue with white coating, and a deep pulse with both *chi* or foot positions especially thready

Therapeutic principles: Supplement the *jing* and boost the qi, warm the kidneys and assist yang

Guiding formula:

Radix Coquitus Rehmanniae (*Shu Di*), 10g
Radix Dioscoreae Oppositae (*Shan Yao*), 30g
Fructus Lycii Chinensis (*Gou Qi*), 15g
Semen Cuscutae (*Tu Si Zi*), 30g
Fructus Ligustri Lucidi (*Nu Zhen Zi*), 20g
Herba Ecliptae Prostratae (*Han Lian Cao*), 15g
Fructus Schizandrae Chinensis (*Wu Wei Zi*), 6g
Ramus Loranthi Seu Visci (*Sang Ji Sheng*), 15g

Colla Cornu Cervi (*Lu Jiao Jiao*), 12g
Herba Epimedii (*Xian Ling Pi*), 15g
Herba Cynomorii Songarici (*Suo Yang*), 12g
Radix Morindae Officinalis (*Ba Ji Tian*), 10g
Fructus Seu Semen Amomi (*Sha Ren*), 6g
Radix Glycyrrhizae (*Gan Cao*)

2. Yin xu huo wang
Yin vacuity, fire effulgent

Pathognomic manifestations: Diminished sperm motility, vexatious heat and especially in the hands and feet, a feeling of unclarity in the head and eyes, a parched mouth but not thirst, a red tongue with no coating, and a thready, rapid pulse

Therapeutic principles: Enrich the kidneys and descend fire

Guiding formula: *Er Xian Tang*

Rhizoma Curculiginis (*Xian Mao*), 6g
Herba Epimedii (*Xian Ling Pi*), 6g
Radix Morindae Officinalis (*Ba Ji Tian*), 6g
Radix Angelicae Sinensis (*Dang Gui*), 6g
Rhizoma Anemarrhenae (*Zhi Mu*), 10g
Cortex Phellodendri (*Huang Bai*), 10g

Jing zi mi du zeng gao
Increased sperm agglutination

Jing zi mi du zeng gao literally means increased or elevated thickening of the sperm. Such thickening is mostly due to agglutination and results in impaired forward progression of the sperm.

Bing yin bing ji
Disease causes, disease mechanisms

Although it is too early to say definitively and categorically, based on preliminary clinical experience, it is surmised that at least one cause of increased sperm agglutination with impaired forward progression is blood stasis.

Bian zheng lun zhi
Treatment based on pattern discrimination

1. *Xue yu*
   ### Blood stasis

Pathognomic manifestations: Increased agglutination of the sperm accompanied by a pale red tongue and a thready, wiry pulse

Therapeutic principles: Activate the blood and transform stasis, assisted by enriching yin, boosting the *jing*, and descending fire as necessary

Guiding formula:

Fructus Liquidambaris Taiwanianae (*Lu Lu Tong*), 30g
Rhizoma Sparganii (*San Leng*), 15g
Rhizoma Curcumae Zedoariae (*E Zhu*), 15g
Semen Pruni Persicae (*Tao Ren*), 15g
Flos Carthami Tinctorii (*Hong Hua*), 10g
Radix Rubrus Paeoniae Lactiflorae (*Chi Shao*), 10g
Rhizoma Ligustici Wallichii (*Chuan Xiong*), 10g
Radix Achyranthis Bidentatae (*Niu Xi*), 30g
Rhizoma Anemarrhenae (*Zhi Mu*), 10g
Cortex Phellodendri (*Huang Bai*), 10g
Fructus Lycii Chinensis (*Gou Qi*), 30g
Fructus Rubi (*Fu Pen Zi*), 30g
Cortex Radicis Moutan (*Dan Pi*), 30g

3

Yin Jing Bing
Diseases of the Penis

Yang wei
Impotence

Impotence is the failure to achieve or maintain an erection sufficient to have unhampered intercourse. According to TCM theory, the penis swells due to an accumulation of both yang qi and yin blood in the penis during sexual excitation.

Bing yin bing ji
Disease causes, disease mechanisms

Impotence can be due to a number of factors, both organic and psychological. Although in ancient times impotence was mostly treated as a kidney disorder, modern TCM theory takes into account the role of the kidneys, liver, spleen, and heart in terms of organ/bowel dysfunction and blood stasis, damp heat, and phlegm turbidity.

As mentioned above, the penis becomes erect when it fills with qi and blood. The testes are called the *wai shen* or external kidneys, and the urethra is one of the two lower portals controlled by the kidneys. Therefore, the genitalia and their function are strongly related to the kidneys. Qi is yang and blood is yin and the kidneys are the root of both true yin and true yang. Therefore, if kidney yang is insufficient, there will not be enough yang qi to fill and raise the penis. Yang qi insufficiency may be due to age, chronic disease, overtaxation and exhaustion, drug use, excessive sex, etc. If kidney yin is insufficient, there may not be enough blood and body fluids to fill the penis until it becomes hard. Kidney yin vacuity may be due to similar causes as well as overthinking, not enough sleep, and persistent restlessness and anxiety.

According to Chinese medicine, the penis is the meeting of the hundred sinews and the sinews are the tissue associated with the liver. In addition, the liver channel encircles the external genitalia. Therefore, almost any problem of the liver can result in impotence. The penis becomes erect not only due to sufficiency of qi flowing to the penis, but also due to a sufficiency of blood filling its sinews. The liver stores the blood; if liver blood becomes vacuous and deficient, there may not be enough blood to fill the penile sinews. If liver qi becomes stagnant and depressed, this may obstruct and constrict the free flow of qi and blood to the genitalia. If the liver is cold, the free flow of qi and blood may also be impeded. In addition, dampness and heat may obstruct the liver channel in the lower burner. Since the liver is called the temperamental organ, many of the psychological causes of impotence are related to liver dysfunction in TCM. However, liver disease may also be due to or complicated by faulty diet, such as overeating sour foods, drinking too much alcohol, and overeating greasy, spicy foods.

Since the spleen and stomach are the postnatal root of qi and blood production, if they become dysfunctional, there may not be enough qi and blood produced to raise the penis and fill its sinews. This may be due to improper or inadequate diet, excessive worry and anxiety, or overtaxation. If the spleen loses its ability to promote the transportation and transformation of body fluids, dampness may accumulate. If it accumulates in the spleen, it will further impede the spleen's ability to generate and transfom the qi and blood. However, dampness, because it is heavy and turbid, tends to percolate down into the lower burner. There it may transform into damp heat or congeal into phlegm. In either case, these yin evils may obstruct what qi and blood there is from gathering in the penis. If damp heat accumulates in the lower burner and obstructs either the liver or kidney channels, this may result in impotence.

The heart is the ruler of the organism but especially rules the blood. The blood which gathers in the penis is sent down to the lower burner by the heart. In addition, erectile potency is also specifically dependent upon heart fire, which connects with the penis and genitalia via the *chong/bao mai*, analogous to the heart's connection with the uterus in females. Vacuity or disturbance of the heart may result in either the heart's loss of command over the blood or loss of communication between heart fire and the genitalia. Further, the heart houses the *shen* and impotence often has a psychological component. When impotence and premature ejaculation are due to fear and timidity regarding sex, this is often diagnosed as heart/gallbladder qi vacuity.

If blood stasis is created, either due to cold, longterm qi stagnation, trauma, longterm obstruction by dampness, phlegm, and/or heat, it may also impede the free flow of qi and blood to the penis. Thus the penis may not be able to become engorged with sufficient qi and blood to become erect. Blood stasis is typically not the main mechanism causing impotence. Rather, it tends to complicate other patterns. Therefore, there is not a separate pattern of blood stasis impotence discussed below, but stasis-transforming, blood-activating medicinals, such as Semen Vaccariae Segetalis (*Wang Bu Liu Xing*), are added to a number of formulas under other patterns.

Bian zheng lun zhi
Treatment based on pattern discrimination

1. *Shen yang kui xu*
Kidney yang deficiency & vacuity

Pathognomic manifestations: Partial erection, decreased sexual desire, lack of erection upon waking, impotence, low back coldness and weakness, soreness and weakness of the knees and legs, tinnitus, dizziness, chilled feet, frequent urination, incontinence, nocturia, tinnitus or deafness, a pale tongue with thin, white coating, and a deep, slow pulse

Therapeutic principles: Supplement the kidneys, strengthen yang, and boost the *jing*

Guiding formulas:

Gui Lu Bu Shen Tang

Colla Cornu Cervi (*Lu Jiao Jiao*), 12g
Colla Plastri Testudinis (*Gui Ban Jiao*), 12g
Fructus Lycii Chinensis (*Gou Qi*), 12g
Herba Cistanchis (*Rou Cong Rong*), 12g
Radix Praeparatus Astragali Seu Hedysari (*Zhi Huang Qi*), 18g
Radix Coquitus Rehmanniae (*Shu Di*), 20g
Herba Epimedii (*Yin Yang Huo*), 9g
Fructus Alpiniae Oxyphyllae (*Yi Zhi Ren*), 9g
Radix Morindae Officinalis (*Ba Ji Tian*), 15g
Actinolitum (*Yang Qi Shi*), 15g

Yang Chuan Yao

Herba Epimedii (*Yin Yang Huo*), 100g
Radix Coquitus Rehmanniae (*Shu Di*), 100g
Actinolitum (*Yang Qi Shi*), 100g
Penis Et Testis Canitis (*Guang Gou Shen*), 100g
Semen Cuscutae (*Tu Si Zi*), 200g
Radix Praeparatus Polygoni Multiflori (*Zhi Shou Wu*), 200g
Fructus Lycii Chinensis (*Gou Qi*), 300g
Cornu Cervi Parvum (*Lu Rong*), 10g
Radix Astragali Seu Hedysari (*Huang Qi*), 50g
Herba Cistanchis (*Rou Cong Rong*), 50g
Sheep penis glue (*Yang Bian Jiao*), 50g
Otter penis glue (*Shui Tiao Bian Jiao*), 20g

Powder the above medicinals and encapsulate, .22g per capsule. Take 2-3 capsules each time, 3 times per day. One course of treatment is 1 month.

Jie Rong San

Gecko (*Ge Jie*), 1 pair
Cornu Cervi Parvum (*Lu Rong*), 20g

Grind into powder and take with wine.

Xin Yang San

Sulphur (*Liu Huang*)
Semen Cnidii Monnieri (*She Chuang Zi*)
Rhizoma Curculiginis Orchoidis (*Xian Mao*)

Grind equal portions of the above medicinals into powder. Take 10g each time, 2 times per day.

She Chi Tang

Semen Cnidii Monnieri (*She Chuang Zi*)
Herba Epimedii (*Yin Yang Huo*)
Actinolitum (*Yang Qi Shi*)
Radix Polygalae Tenuifoliae (*Yuan Zhi*)
Fructus Schizandrae Chinensis (*Wu Wei Zi*)

Additions:

For severe cold, add Cortex Cinnamomi (*Rou Gui*) and Radix Praeparatus Aconiti Carmichaeli (*Fu Zi*).

For spermatorrhea and premature ejaculation, add Fructus Rosae Laevigatae (*Jin Ying Zi*) and Ootheca Manitis (*Sang Piao Xiao*).

Zhuang Yang Chi Wei Wan

Radix Codonopsis Pilosulae (*Lu Dang Shen*), 12g
Rhizoma Atractylodis Macrocephalae (*Bai Zhu*), 12g
Fructus Lycii Chinensis (*Gou Qi*), 12g
Cordyceps Chinensis (*Dong Chong Xiao Cao*), 12g
Radix Coquitus Rehmanniae (*Shu Di*), 12g
Actinolitum (*Yang Chi Shi*), 12g
Semen Allii Tuberosi (*Jiu Cai Zi*), 12g
Carapax Amydae (*Bie Jia*), 30g
Plastrum Testudinis (*Gui Ban*), 30g
Cortex Eucommiae Ulmoidis (*Du Zhong*), 9g
Herba Cynomorii Songarici (*Suo Yang*), 9g
Herba Epimedii (*Xian Ling Pi*), 9g
Radix Angelicae Sinensis (*Dang Gui Shen*), 9g
Radix Dipsaci (*Chuan Xu Duan*), 9g
Herba Cistanchis (*Rou Cong Rong*), 9g
Fructus Psoraleae Corylifoliae (*Po Gu Zhi*), 9g
Placenta Hominis (*Zi He Che*), 9g
Radix Praeparatus Glycyrrhizae (*Zhi Gan Cao*), 9g
Semen Cuscutae (*Tu Si Zi*), 15g

Grind into powder and make into pills. Take 3-6 pills each time, 3 times per day. One month is 1 course of treatment.

2. Shen yin xu
Kidney yin vacuity

Pathognomic manifestations: Impotence, dizziness, tinnitus, soreness and weakness of the low back and knees, heat in the five centers, a dry mouth and parched throat, night sweats, scanty sleep and excessive dreams, constipation, a red tongue with a scant coating, and a thready, rapid pulse

Therapeutic principles: Supplement the kidneys and enrich yin, repress yang and generate fluids

Guiding formulas:

Di Long Tang

Lumbricus Terrestris (*Di Long*), 10g
Radix Dioscoreae Oppositae (*Shan Yao*), 10g
Fructus Corni Officinalis (*Shan Yu Rou*), 10g
Semen Cuscutae (*Tu Si Zi*), 10g
Tuber Asparagi Cochinensis (*Tian Dong*), 10g
Fructus Lycii Chinensis (*Gou Qi Zi*), 10g
Colla Plastri Testudinis (*Gui Ban Jiao*), 10g
Radix Coquitus Rehmanniae (*Shu Di*), 12g
Concha Ostreae (*Sheng Mu Li*), 12g
Cortex Radicis Moutan (*Dan Pi*), 6g

Additions & subtractions:

For yin vacuity with stirring of fire, add Rhizoma Anemarrhenae
(*Zhi Mu*) and Cortex Phellodendri (*Huang Bai*). Use Radix
Rehmanniae (*Sheng Di*) to replace Radix Coquitus Rehmanniae
(*Shu Di*), and subtract Fructus Lycii Chinensis and Semen
Cuscutae.

For liver qi stagnation, add Cortex Albizziae Julibrissinis (*He Huan
Pi*).

For heart spirit not calm, add Semen Zizyphi Spinosae (*Suan Zao
Ren*) and Radix Polygalae Tenuifoliae (*Yuan Zhi*).

For damp heat pouring downward, add Rhizoma Dioscoreae Bixie
(*Bi Xie*) and Semen Plantaginis (*Che Qian Zi*).

For spermatorrhea, add Stamen Nelumbinis Nuciferae (*Lian Xu*)
and Fructus Rosae Laevigatae (*Jin Ying Zi*).

Zi Yin Chi Wei Tang

Radix Coquitus Rehmanniae (*Shu Di*), 20-40g
Radix Polygoni Multiflori (*Shou Wu*), 40g
Fructus Lycii Chinensis (*Gou Qi Zi*), 20g

Radix Dioscoreae Oppositae (*Shan Yao*), 15g
Actinolitum (*Yang Qi Shi*), 15-30g, wrap in cheesecloth
Herba Epimedii (*Yin Yang Huo*), 5-10g
Herba Ephedrae Sinicae (*Ma Huang*), 1-3g
Pulvis Testis Et Penis Canitis (*Huang Gou Shen Fen*), 1g

3. *Shen yin yang liang xu*
Kidney yin & yang dual vacuity

Pathognomic manifestations: Impotence, failure to maintain an erection, low back pain, soreness and weakness of the low back and knees, dizziness, tinnitus, night sweats, excessive spontaneous sweating, chilly coldness of the hands and feet or heat in the centers of the hands and feet, a red tongue tip with a thin, white coating, and a thready, rapid, forceless pulse

Therapeutic principles: Enrich kidney yin and supplement kidney yang

Guiding formula: *Yi Jing Zhuang Yang Tang*

Radix Dioscoreae Oppositae (*Shan Yao*), 20g
Radix Coquitus Rehmanniae (*Shu Di*), 20g
Fructus Lycii Chinensis (*Gou Qi*), 20g
Fructus Corni Officinalis (*Shan Zhu Yu*), 20g
Sclerotium Poriae Cocoris (*Fu Ling*), 15g
Herba Cistanchis (*Rou Cong Rong*), 15g
Herba Cynomorii Songarici (*Suo Yang*), 15g
Radix Morindae Officinalis (*Ba Ji Tian*), 15g
Radix Panacis Ginseng (*Ren Shen*), 15g
Semen Praeparatus Zizyphi Spinosae (*Zhi Zao Ren*), 15g
Semen Cuscutae (*Tu Si Zi*), 15g
Tuber Asparagi Cochinensis (*Tian Dong*), 10g
Radix Glycyrrhizae (*Gan Cao*), 10g

4. *Shi re xia zhu shen jing*
Damp heat pouring down into the kidney channel

Pathognomic manifestations: Impotence, yellow, frequent, difficult, painful urination, possible itching, dampness, and inflammation of the genitalia, a red tongue with yellow, slimy coating, and a slippery, rapid pulse

Therapeutic principles: Clear heat and disinhibit dampness from the kidney channel

Guiding formulas:

Bi Xie Fen Qing Yin (see above) plus

Zhi Bai Di Huang Wan (see above) plus

Si Mao San

Cortex Phellodendri (*Huang Bai*)
Rhizoma Atractylodis (*Cang Zhu*)
Radix Achyranthis Bidentatae (*Niu Xi*)

Wu Ling San (see above) plus

Cortex Phellodendri (*Huang Bai*)
Talcum (*Hua Shi*)
Caulis Akebiae Mutong (*Mu Tong*)
Semen Coicis Lachryma-jobi (*Yi Yi Ren*)

5. *Gan yu qi zhi*
Liver depression, qi stagnation

Pathognomic manifestations: Irritability, depression, chest oppression, flank pain, lower abdominal pain, pain associated with the scrotal region, and a wiry pulse

Therapeutic principles: Course the liver, resolve depression, and regulate the qi

Guiding formulas:

Xiao Yao San

Radix Bupleuri (*Chai Hu*)
Radix Angelicae Sinensis (*Dang Gui*)
Radix Albus Paeoniae Lactiflorae (*Bai Shao*)
Rhizoma Atractylodis Macrocephalae (*Bai Zhu*)
Sclerotium Poriae Cocoris (*Fu Ling*)
Radix Praeparatus Glycyrrhizae (*Zhi Gan Cao*)
Herba Menthae (*Bo He*)
Rhizoma Recens Zingiberis (*Sheng Jiang*)

Chai Hu Shu Gan Tang

Radix Bupleuri (*Chai Hu*)
Radix Albus Paeoniae Lactiflorae (*Bai Shao*)
Fructus Citri Seu Ponciri (*Zhi Qiao*)
Rhizoma Ligustici Wallichii (*Chuan Xiong*)
Rhizoma Cyperi Rotundi (*Xiang Fu*)
Radix Glycyrrhizae (*Gan Cao*)

Kai Yu Chong Yu Tang (see above)

Si Ni San

Radix Bupleuri (*Chai Hu*)
Fructus Immaturus Citri Seu Ponciri (*Zhi Shi*)
Radix Albus Paeoniae Lactiflorae (*Bai Shao*)
Radix Glycyrrhizae (*Gan Cao*)

Gan Mai Da Zao Tang

Radix Glycyrrhizae (*Gan Cao*), 9-12g
Fructus Levis Tritici (*Fu Xiao Mai*), 30-50g
Fructus Zizyphi Jujubae (*Da Zao*), 10-15 pieces

Li Qi Tong Tang

Semen Citri (*Ju He*), 10g
Radix Bupleuri (*Chai Hu*), 10g
Fructus Citri Seu Ponciri (*Zhi Ke*), 10g
Radix Albus Paeoniae Lactiflorae (*Bai Shao*), 10g
Herba Lycopodii (*Shen Jin Cao*), 15g
Semen Cnidii Monnieri (*She Chuang Zi*), 12g
Semen Allii Tuberosi (*Jiu Cai Zi*), 12g
Bulbus Allii (*Xie Bai*), 9g
Semen Vaccariae Segetalis (*Wang Bu Liu Xing*), 9g

6. Gan jing shi re
Damp heat in the liver channel

Pathognomic manifestations: Impotence, vexation, easily angered, possible chest and flank distention and fullness, irascibility, lack of strength, excessive dreams, dizziness, tinnitus, numbness of the extremities, edema, yellow urine, loose stools, a slightly fat tongue with teeth indentations, and a wiry, rapid pulse

Therapeutic principles: Course the liver and resolve depression, clear heat and disinhibit dampness

Guiding formulas:

Long Dan Xie Gan Tang (see above)

Qing Gan Li Shi Tang

Cortex Phellodendri (*Huang Bai*), 12g
Radix Scutellariae Baicalensis (*Huang Qin*), 12g
Herba Dianthi (*Qu Mai*), 12g
Herba Polygoni Avicularis (*Bian Xu*), 12g
Talcum (*Hua Shi*), 12g
Fructus Gardeniae Jasminoidis (*Zhi Zi*), 9g
Semen Plantaginis (*Che Qian Zi*), 9g
Caulis Akebiae Mutong (*Mu Tong*), 6g
Radix Bupleuri (*Chai Hu*), 6g

Herba Artemesiae Capillaris (*Yin Chen*), 10g
Semen Cnidii Monnieri (*She Chuan Zi*), 10g
Semen Vaccariae Segetalis (*Wang Bu Liu Xing*), 10g
Herba Lycopodii (*Shen Jin Cao*), 15g

Shu Gan Qing Li Tang

Radix Bupleuri (*Chai Hu*), 9g
Fructus Citri Seu Ponciri (*Zhi Ke*), 9g
Rhizoma Atractylodis (*Cang Zhu*), 9g
Cortex Phellodendri (*Huang Bai*), 10g
Rhizoma Anemarrhenae (*Zhi Mu*), 10g
Radix Salviae Miltiorrhizae (*Dan Shen*), 12g
Radix Angelicae Sinensis (*Dang Gui*), 12g
Fructus Liquidambaris Taiwanianae (*Lu Lu Tong*), 12g
Radix Achyranthis Bidentatae (*Niu Xi*), 15g
Rhizoma Imperatae Cylindricae (*Bai Mao Geng*), 20g
Semen Coicis Lachryma-jobi (*Yi Yi Ren*), 20g
Radix Gentianae Scabrae (*Long Dan Cao*), 18g

Unnamed formula:

Radix Bupleuri (*Chai Hu*)
Caulis Perillae Frutescentis (*Su Geng*)
Herba Agastachis Seu Pogostemi (*Huo Xiang*)
Radix Angelicae Pubescentis (*Du Huo*)
Semen Alpiniae Katsumadai (*Cao Dou*)
Semen Plantaginis (*Che Qian Zi*)
Fructus Gardeniae Jasminoidis (*Zhi Zi*)
Radix Scutellariae Baicalensis (*Huang Qin*)
Radix Gentianae Scabrae (*Long Dan Cao*)
Radix Et Rhizoma Rhei (*Da Huang*) treated with vinegar

7. Gan han
Liver cold

Pathognomic manifestations: Impotence, cold feeling in the testicles and scrotum, cold feeling in the lower body in general, stuffiness and distention in the chest and abdomen, a pale face, and a deep, tight pulse

Therapeutic principles: Warm the liver and disinhibit the qi

Guiding formulas:

Nuan Gan Jian

Radix Angelicae Sinensis (*Dang Gui*), 6-9g
Fructus Lycii Chinensis (*Gou Qi*), 9g
Fructus Foeniculi Vulgaris (*Xiao Hui Xiang*), 6g
Cortex Cinnamomi (*Rou Gui*), 3-6g
Radix Linderae Strychnifoliae (*Wu Yao*), 6g
Lignum Aquilariae Agallochae (*Chen Xiang*), 3g
Sclerotium Poriae Cocoris (*Fu Ling*), 6g
Rhizoma Recens Zingiberis (*Sheng Jiang*), 3-5 slices

Nuan Gan Wen Jing Tang

Fructus Foeniculi Vulgaris (*Xiao Hui Xiang*), 15 g
Amethystum (*Zi Shi Ying*), 15g
Semen Citri (*Ju He*), 10g
Semen Litchi Chinensis (*Li Zhi He*), 10g
Sclerotium Poriae Cocoris (*Fu Ling*), 10g
Semen Allii Tuberosi (*Jiu Cai Zi*), 10g
Cortex Cinnamomi (*Rou Gui*), 10g
Radix Morindae Officinalis (*Ba Ji Tian*), 6g
Herba Epimedii (*Yin Yang Huo*), 6g
Semen Vaccariae Segetalis (*Wang Bu Liu Xing*), 6g
Herba Lycopodii (*Shen Jin Cao*), 12g

8. Gan xue yin xu
Liver blood & yin vacuity

Pathognomic manifestations: Impotence, emotional upset, anger, depression, frequent sighing, dizziness, blurred vision, fatigue, a red tongue with a scant coating, and a thready, wiry pulse

Therapeutic principles: Nourish yin and soften the liver

Guiding formulas:

Shao Yao Gan Cao Tang Jia Wei

Radix Albus Paeoniae Lactiflorae (*Bai Shao*), 15g
Radix Praeparatus Glycyrrhizae (*Zhi Gan Cao*), 15g
Radix Angelicae Sinensis (*Dang Gui*), 12g
Radix Coquitus Rehmanniae (*Shu Di*), 12g
Rhizoma Polygonati (*Huang Jing*), 9g
Fructus Corni Officinalis (*Shan Yu Rou*), 9g
Fructus Schizandrae Chinensis (*Wu Wei Zi*), 9g
Fructus Lycii Chinensis (*Gou Qi Zi*), 6g

Rou Gan Chi Wei Tang

Radix Astragali Seu Hedysari (*Huang Qi*), 15g
Radix Albus Paeoniae Lactiflorae (*Bai Shao*), 15g
Radix Puerariae Lobatae (*Ge Geng*), 15g
Flouritum (*Zi Shi Ying*), 15g
Radix Praeparatus Polygoni Multiflori (*Zhi Shou Wu*), 20g
Radix Dioscoreae Oppositae (*Shan Yao*), 20g
Fructus Lycii Chinensis (*Gou Qi Zi*), 10g
Semen Allii Tuberosi (*Jiu Cai Zi*), 10g
Radix Morindae Officinalis (*Ba Ji Tian*), 10g
Herba Lycopodii (*Shen Jin Cao*), 10g
Semen Cuscutae (*Tu Si Zi*), 12g

9. Xin dan qi xu
Heart/gallbladder qi vacuity

Pathognomic manifestations: Impotence, spermatorrhea, premature ejaculation, heart palpitations, heart not calm, easily frightened, timidity, fear of sex, a pale tongue with white coating, and a wiry, thready pulse

Therapeutic principles: Nourish the heart and calm the spirit, supplement the *jing* and assist the gallbladder

Guiding formulas:

Da Bu Yuan Jian

Radix Coquitus Rehmanniae (*Shu Di*), 20g
Fructus Corni Officinalis (*Shan Zhu Yu*), 15g
Radix Dioscoreae Oppositae (*Shan Yao*), 15g
Fructus Lycii Chinensis (*Gou Qi Zi*), 20g
Cortex Eucommiae Ulmoidis (*Du Zhong*), 15g
Radix Codonopsis Pilosulae (*Dang Shen*), 15g
Radix Glycyrrhizae (*Gan Cao*), 10g
Radix Angelicae Sinensis (*Dang Gui*), 15g

Ren Re San

Semen Biotae Orientalis (*Bai Zi Ren*), 15g
Radi Coquitus Rehmanniae (*Shu Di*), 20g
Fructus Lycii Chinensis (*Gou Qi Zi*), 25g
Fructus Corni Officinalis (*Shan Zhu Yu*), 15g
Fructus Schizandrae Chinensis (*Wu Wei Zi*), 15g
Radix Panacis Ginseng (*Ren Shen*), 15g
Sclerotium Pararadicis Poriae Cocoris (*Fu Shen*), 15g
Flos Chrysanthemi Morifolii (*Ju Hua*), 10g
Fructus Citri Seu Ponciri (*Zhi Qiao*), 10g
Cortex Cinnamomi (*Gui Xin*), 5g

Powder the above ingredients. Take 9g each time, 2 times per day. Swallow with wine.

10. *Pi wei xu rou*
Spleen/stomach vacuity weakness

Pathognomic manifestations: Impotence accompanied by digestive complaints such as loss of appetite, diarrhea and loose stools, weakness of the entire body, lack of strength in the extremities, shortness of breath, dizziness, soreness and weakness of the low back and knees, a pale tongue with a thin, white coating, and a minute, weak, forceless pulse

Therapeutic principles: Supplement the center and boost the qi

Guiding formulas:

Bu Zhong Yi Qi Tang

Radix Astragali Seu Hedysari (*Huang Qi*)
Radix Panacis Ginseng (*Ren Shen*)
Rhizoma Atractylodis Macrocephalae (*Bai Zhu*)
Radix Praeparatus Glycyrrhizae (*Zhi Gan Cao*)
Radix Angelicae Sinensis (*Dang Gui*)
Rhizoma Cimicifugae (*Sheng Ma*)
Radix Bupleuri (*Chai Hu*)
Pericarpium Citri Reticulatae (*Chen Pi*)

Ren Shen Yang Rong Tang

Radix Angelicae Sinensis (*Dang Gui*), 15g
Radix Coquitus Rehmanniae (*Shu Di*), 15g
Radix Albus Paeoniae Lactiflorae (*Bai Shao*), 15g
Radix Panacis Ginseng (*Ren Shen*), 15g
Rhizoma Atractylodis Macrocephalae (*Bai Zhu*), 15g
Sclerotium Poriae Cocoris (*Fu Ling*), 15g
Radix Astragali Seu Hedysari (*Huang Qi*), 20g
Cortex Cinnamomi (*Rou Gui*), 5g
Fructus Schizandrae Chinensis (*Wu Wei Zi*), 10g
Pericarpium Citri Reticulatae (*Chen Pi*), 10g
Radix Polygalae Tenuifoliae (*Yuan Zhi*), 10g

Radix Praeparatus Glycyrrhizae (*Zhi Gan Cao*), 10g
Rhizoma Recens Zingiberis (*Sheng Jiang*), 3 slices
Fructus Zizyphi Jujubae (*Da Zao*), 4 pieces

Huang Qi Jian Zhong Tang

Radix Astragali Seu Hedysari (*Huang Qi*), 30g
Radix Albus Paeoniae Lactiflorae (*Bai Shao*), 20g
Cortex Cinnamomi (*Gui Pi*), 15g
Radix Glycyrrhizae (*Gan Cao*), 10g
Maltose (*Yi Tang*), 30g

11. Pi xu tan shi
Spleen vacuity, phlegm dampness

Pathognomic manifestations: Impotence, obesity, phlegmatic cough, dizziness, nausea, stuffy chest, a heavy sensation in the body, inhibited urination, a pale tongue with a slimy coating, and a slippery pulse

Therapeutic principles: Strengthen the spleen and supplement the qi, transform phlegm and eliminate dampness

Guiding formula: Er Chen Tang

Rhizoma Pinelliae Ternatae (*Ban Xia*)
Pericarpium Citri Reticulatae (*Chen Pi*)
Sclerotium Poriae Cocoris (*Fu Ling*)
Radix Glycyrrhizae (*Gan Cao*)

12. Xin pi xu kui
Heart/spleen vacuity & deficiency

Pathognomic manifestations: Impotence, heart palpitations, heart not calm, scanty sleep, excessive dreams, diminished appetite, stuffy epigastrium, lack of strength in the four limbs, loose stools, slight edema, a pale tongue with scant coating, and a deep, weak pulse

Therapeutic principles: Supplement and boost the spleen and heart, assist yang and raise atony

Guiding formulas:

Gui Pi Tang

Radix Codonopsis Pilosulae (*Dang Shen*), 30g
Rhizoma Atractylodis Macrocephalae (*Bai Zhu*), 15g
Sclerotium Poriae Cocoris (*Fu Ling*), 15g
Radix Praeparatus Glycyrrhizae (*Zhi Gan Cao*), 10g
Radix Praeparatus Polygalae Tenuifoliae (*Zhi Yuan Zhi*), 15g
Semen Zizyphi Spinosae (*Suan Zao Ren*), 15g
Radix Astragali Seu Hedysari (*Huang Qi*), 20g
Arillus Euphoriae Longanae (*Long Yan Rou*), 15g
Radix Angelicae Sinensis (*Dang Gui*), 15g
Radix Saussureae Seu Vladimiriae (*Mu Xiang*), 10g
Fructus Zizyphi Jujubae (*Da Zao*), 3 pieces
Rhizoma Recens Zingiberis (*Sheng Jiang*), 3 slices

Qi Fu Yin

Rhizoma Atractylodis Macrocephalae (*Bai Zhu*), 15g
Radix Polygalae Tenuifoliae (*Yuan Zhi*), 15g
Radix Coquitus Rehmanniae (*Shu Di*), 25g
Fructus Zizyphi Spinosae (*Zao Ren*), 15g
Radix Panacis Ginseng (*Ren Shen*), 15g
Radix Glycyrrhizae (*Gan Cao*), 5g
Radix Angelicae Sinensis (*Dang Gui*), 20g

13. *Wai gan shi re*
   External attack of damp heat

Pathognomic manifestations: Impotence or persistent erection, headache, a heavy sensation in the body, stuffy chest, lower abdominal distention, dampness of the external genitalia, difficult urination, a thick, white or slimy, yellow tongue coating, and a sodden, fast, floating pulse

Therapeutic principles: Clear heat and disinhibit dampness

Guiding formulas:

San Ren Tang (see above)

Qiang Huo Shen Shi Tang

Radix Et Rhizoma Notopterygii (*Qiang Huo*)
Radix Angelicae Pubescentis (*Du Huo*)
Radix Et Rhizoma Ligustici Sinensis (*Gao Ben*)
Radix Ledebouriellae Sesloidis (*Fang Feng*)
Rhizoma Ligustici Wallichii (*Chuan Xiong*)
Fructus Viticis (*Man Jing Zi*)
Radix Praeparatus Glycyrrhizae (*Zhi Gan Cao*)

Si Miao San

Cortex Phellodendri (*Huang Bai*), 9g
Rhizoma Atractylodis (*Cang Zhu*), 12g
Radix Achyranthis Bidentatae (*Huai Niu Xi*), 9g
Semen Coicis Lachryma-jobi (*Yi Yi Ren*), 9g

Acupuncture/moxibustion therapy

Kidney vacuity

1. *Zhong Ji* (CV 3), *Guan Yuan* (CV 4), *Qi Hai* (CV 6), *Shen Shu* (Bl 23), and *Ming Men* (GV 4)

2. *Guan Yuan* (CV 4), *Zhong Wan* (CV 12), *Shen Shu* (Bl 23), *San Yin Jiao* (Sp 6), and *Bai Hui* (GV 20) as the main points, supplemented as needed by *Yin Tang* (M-HN-3), *Qi Hai* (CV 6), *Da Zhui* (GV 14), and *Ming Men* (GV 4)

Heart/spleen dual vacuity

Xin Shu (Bl 15), *Nei Guan* (Per 6), *San Yin Jiao* (Sp 6), *Guan Yuan* (CV 4), and *Shen Shu* (Bl 23) as the main points plus *Zu San Li* (St 36), *Da Zhui* (GV 14), and *Yin Tang* (M-HN-3)

Damp heat pouring downwards

Li Gou (Liv 5), *Guan Yuan* (CV 4), *San Yin Jiao* (Sp 6), and *Yang Ling Quan* (GB 34) plus *Shen Shu* (Bl 23), *Da Zhu* (Bl 10), *Dan Shu* (Bl 19), and *Tai Chong* (Liv 3)

Combined acupuncture & moxibustion treatment

Needle *Zhong Ji* (CV 3), *Guan Yuan* (CV 4), and *Tai Xi* (Ki 3) and then moxa 3-5 cones; moxa indirectly *Hui Yin* (CV 1) with a moxa pole.

Ear acupuncture treatment

Kidneys, Subcortex, External Genitalia

Yang qiang
Persistent erection

Yang qiang means yang striving or straining. It refers to persistent erection or priapism. This may last from a couple of hours to a couple of days or even a couple of months and is often combined with penile pain. According to modern Western medicine, priapism may be due to either vascular or neurological abnormalities. It may also be secondary to prolonged sexual activity; leukemia or other blood dyscrasias; pelvic hematoma or neoplasm; cerebrospinal disease, such as syphilis or tumor; or infection and inflammation of the male urogenital organs, such as prostatitis, urethritis, and cystitis complicated by bladder stones.

Bing yin bing ji
Disease causes, disease mechanisms

Abnormal persistent erection may be due to any of four reasons. First, evil dampness and heat may pour down into the lower burner engorging the penis. Although these are evil qi, they may, nonetheless, fill up the penis pathologically analogous to how righteous yang qi and yin fluids fill up the penis ordinarily. The causes of dampness and heat have been discussed above. Damp heat is most often encountered in young patients.

Secondly, yin vacuity may give rise to exuberance and reckless stirring of ministerial fire. In this case, the evil heat engorging the penis is vacuity heat. In this case, excessive sexual desire will also be experienced. Vacuity heat persistent erection is most often encountered in older patients due to the natural consumption and decline of kidney yin attendant with aging.

Third, liver/gallbladder replete heat may cause excessive engorgement of yang qi in the penis. This is most often due to emotional frustration leading to qi stagnation which, in turn, transforms into depressive heat. In this case, instead of this heat rising upward, it travels down along the liver channel to the genitalia, there to accumulate and engorge the penis. Liver heat is commonly encountered in young and middle-aged patients.

And fourth, blood stasis may obstruct the channels leading into and away from the penis. Although blood stasis can also cause impotence or failure of the penis to engorge, in other cases, once the penis has engorged, blood stasis may obstruct the flow of yang qi and yin fluids out of the penis, thus maintaining erection. When this occurs, it may be as a complication of one of the two scenarios above or as the main disease mechanism in and of itself. When blood stasis plays a part in persistent erection or priapism, Western medicine often detects the presence of neoplasms.

Bian zheng lun zhi
Treatment based on pattern discrimination

1. Shi re xia zhu
Damp heat pouring downward

Pathognomic manifestations: Persistent erection, lower abdominal distention, damp, painful scrotum and testes, difficult urination, a thick, yellow tongue coating, and a wiry, rapid, slippery pulse

Therapeutic principles: Clear heat and disinhibit dampness

Guiding formula: Long Dan Xie Gan Tang (see above)

2. Yin shi yang shi
Yin vacuity, yang repletion

Pathognomic manifestations: Persistent erection, tinnitus, dizziness, insomnia, night sweats, restlessness, palpitations, poor memory, blurred vision, polyuria, nocturia, a red tongue, and a thready, rapid pulse

Therapeutic principles: Nourish yin, descend and clear fire, and soften the hard

Guiding formulas:

Zhi Bai Di Huang Wan (see above)

Da Bu Yin Wan (see above)

Shao Yao Gan Cao Tang

Radix Albus Paeoniae Lactiflorae (*Shao Yao*)
Radix Praeparatus Glycyrrhizae (*Zhi Gan Cao*)

To these three formulas, add medicinals to activate the blood, open the channels, and soften the hard as necessary.

3. *Gan dan shi huo*
   Liver/gallbladder replete fire

Pathognomic manifestations: Persistent engorgement of the penis typically accompanied by pain, easily angered, dizziness, tinnitus, red face, bitter taste in the mouth, dry throat, a red tongue with a dry, yellow coating, and a wiry, forceful pulse

Therapeutic principles: Clear and discharge liver fire, assisted by enriching yin and softening the hard

Guiding formula: *Dang Gui Long Hui Tang*

Radix Angelicae Sinensis (*Dang Gui*), 10g
Radix Gentianae Scabrae (*Long Dan Cao*), 15g
Herba Aloes (*Lu Hui*), 6g
Radix Scutellariae Baicalensis (*Huang Qin*), 5g
Rhizoma Coptidis Chinensis (*Huang Lian*), 5g
Cortex Phellodendri (*Huang Bai*), 5g
Radix Et Rhizoma Rhei (*Da Huang*), 5g
Radix Saussureae Seu Vladimiriae (*Mu Xiang*), 3g
Rhizoma Ligustici Wallichii (*Chuan Xiong*), 10g
Radix Bupleuri (*Chai Hu*), 10g
Pulvis Indigonis (*Qing Dai*), 5g

4. *Xue yu*
   Blood stasis

Pathognomic manifestations: Persistent erection, pain in the scrotum and testicles, painful, difficult urination, lower abdominal spasm, red spots on the tongue with a yellow coating, and a deep, wiry pulse

Therapeutic principles: Activate the blood and transform stasis

Guiding formula: *Xue Fu Zhu Yu Tang* (see above)

Yin jing tong
Penile pain

Pain in the penis may be either localized to one spot or diffuse, encompassing the entire penis.

Bing yin bing ji
Disease causes, disease mechanisms

According to TCM theory, penile pain is mostly due to cold contraction of the channel. Cold causes blockage to the qi and blood which then accumulates behind this blockage. This accumulation distends and puts pressure upon the surrounding tissue, and thus pain is produced. This cold may be either vacuous or replete, and often is a combination of both where kidney yang vacuity allows for invasion of external cold. In some rare cases, penile pain may also be due to injury due to heat.

Bian zheng lun zhi
Treatment based on pattern discrimination

1. Han yu zu jing
Cold stasis obstructing the channels

Pathognomic manifestations: Dull pain in the penis with scrotal retraction, coldness of the limbs, possible fatigue, a pale, possibly flabby tongue with a thin, white coating, and a deep, thready, slow pulse

Therapeutic principles: Dispel cold and open the channels

Guiding formula: Ma Huang Xi Xin Fu Zi Tang Jia Wei

Herba Ephedrae Sinicae (*Ma Huang*)
Radix Praeparatus Aconiti Carmichaeli (*Fu Zi*)
Herba Cum Radice Asari Seiboldi (*Xi Xin*)
Rhizoma Praeparata Zingiberis (*Pao Jiang*)
Rhizoma Ligustici Wallichii (*Chuan Xiong*)

Semen Pruni Persicae (*Tao Ren*)

Acupuncture/moxibustion therapy

Needle *Guan Yuan* (CV 4) and *San Yin Jiao* (Sp 6) with strong
stimulation until the sensation is propagated to the genitalia.

Yin jing ai
Penile cancer

Penile cancer is called *yin jing ai* in modern Chinese. Its traditional
name is *shen yan*. *Shen yan* literally means kidney rock. The word
"rock" is commonly used for a hard cancerous tumor in Chinese
medicine. However, the word "kidney" is used in this case because
the penis is traditionally associated with the kidneys. For instance,
the testes are called the "external kidneys". According to modern
Western medicine, penile cancer is most common in uncircumcised
males who practice poor local hygiene. Typically the tumor forms
below the foreskin on the glans or head of the penis. Mostly penile
cancer occurs in middle-aged or older men. In some cases, penile
cancer may develop out of venereal warts. In this case, the tumors
are acanthotic (like cauliflower) and so are called *fan hua shen yan*
or cauliflower kidney rocks. Modern Western medicine considers
penile cancer refractory to standard therapies, such as chemothera-
py and radiotherapy.

Bing yin bing ji
Disease causes, disease mechanisms

Traditionally, penile cancer is primarily believed to be due to
dampness and heat, stasis, and toxins. We have discussed the cases
and mechanisms of the first three above. Toxins refers to
especially virulent evils, often due to excessive heat or long-term
brewing of dampness and heat.

Bian zheng lun zhi
Treatment based on pattern discrimination

1. *Shi re yu du*
Damp heat, stasis, & toxins

Pathognomic manifestations: A painful, swollen mass on the external genitalia accompanied by lower abdominal distention, frequent, dribbling urination, fever, dry mouth with a desire to drink, a yellow tongue coating, and a rapid pulse

Therapeutic principles: Clear heat and disinhibit dampness, resolve toxins and transform stasis

Guiding formulas:

Ju Zao Wan

Flos Chrysanthemi (*Ju Hua*), 100g
Herba Sargassi (*Hai Zao*), 100g
Rhizoma Sparganii (*San Leng*), 100g
Rhizoma Curcumae Zedoariae (*E Zhu*), 100g
Radix Codonopsis Pilosulae (*Dang Shen*), 100g
Radix Astragali Seu Hedysari (*Huang Qi*), 100g
Flos Lonicerae Japonicae (*Yin Hua*), 100g
Radix Sophorae Subprostratae (*Shan Dou Geng*), 100g
Bulbus Shancigu (*Shan Ci Gu*), 100g
Radix Rhapontici Seu Echinopsis (*Lou Lu*), 100g
Radix Arnebiae Seu Lithospermae (*Zi Cao*), 25g
Rhizoma Coptidis Chinensis (*Huang Lian*), 25g
Semen Strychnotis (*Ma Qian Zi*), 50g
Scolopendra Subspinipes (*Wu Gong*), 50g
Radix Et Rhizoma Rhei (*Da Huang*), 15g

Grind the above ingredients and make into small pills. Take 25-30 pills each time, 3 times per day 1 hour after meals.

Zhi Bai Di Huang Wan He San Miao Wan Jia Jian

Radix Rehmanniae (*Sheng Di*), 9g
Radix Coquitus Rehmanniae (*Shu Di*), 9g
Rhizoma Anemarrhenae (*Zhi Mu*), 9g
Cortex Phellodendri (*Huang Bai*), 9g
Cortex Radicis Moutan (*Dan Pi*), 9g
Fructus Corni Officinalis (*Shan Zhu Yu*), 9g
Sclerotium Poriae Cocoris (*Fu Ling*), 12g
Rhizoma Atractylodis (*Cang Zhu*), 12g
Carapax Amydae (*Bie Jia*), 15g
Radix Gentianae Scabrae (*Long Dan Cao*), 4.5g
Semen Coicis Lachryma-jobi (*Yi Yi Ren*), 30g
Radix Salviae Miltiorrhizae (*Dan Shen*), 30g

Additions:

For metastasis to the lymph nodes of the groin, add Spica Prunellae Vulgaris (*Xia Gu Cao*), 9g, and Sargassum (*Ha Zao*), 9g.

For exudation and weeping, add Rhizoma Dioscoreae Bixie (*Bi Xie*), 12g, Herba Polypodii Hastati (*Qi Xing Cao*), 30g, and Radix Glycyrrhizae (*Gan Cao*), 4.5g

For qi and blood vacuity, add Radix Codonopsis Pilosulae (*Dang Shen*), 9g, Radix Astragali Seu Hedysari (*Huang Qi*), 9g, and Rhizoma Atractylodis Macrocephalae (*Bai Zhu*), 9g.

For yin vacuity, add Herba Ecliptae Prostratae (*Han Lian Cao*), 15g, and Fructus Ligustri Lucidi (*Nu Zhen Zi*), 15g.

For yang vacuity, add *You Gui Wan* (see above).

For swelling of the lower extremities, add Semen Phaseoli Calcarati (*Chi Xiao Dou*), 30g, and Semen Benincasae Hispidae (*Dong Gua Ren*), 15g.

Yin jing lao
Tuberculosis of the penis

Tuberculosis, although on the rise in the United States, is still more common in the People's Republic of China. It is possible for the penis to be the site of direct infection of the tuberculosis bacillus, thus causing penile tuberculosis. It is also possible for penile tuberculosis to result secondarily from tubercular infection of the lungs and/or kidneys. In TCM, penile tuberculosis is known as *yin jing lao* which translates as penile taxation, *i.e.*, consumption.

Bing yin bing ji
Disease causes, disease mechanisms

This disease is most commonly seen in patients with a righteous qi insufficiency. This weakness and deficiency predisposes such patients to invasion by the tuberculosis bacillus. Like most *xu lao* or vacuity taxation diseases, yin vacuity is at the root of this condition. This yin vacuity may be due to congenital insufficiency or taxation including sexual taxation, drug use, poor diet, etc.

Bian zheng lun zhi
Treatment based on pattern discrimination

1. *Yin xu huo dong*
Yin vacuity, stirring of fire

Pathognomic manifestations: Ulceration of the penis, a dry mouth, yellow urine, a red tongue, and a thready, rapid pulse

Therapeutic principles: Nourish yin and descend fire

Guiding formula: *Zhi Bai Di Huang Wan Jia Jian*

Radix Rehmanniae (*Sheng Di*), 12g
Plastrum Praeparatum Testudinis (*Zhi Gui Ban*), 18g
Fructus Corni Officinalis (*Shan Yu Rou*), 5g

Rhizoma Anemarrhenae (*Zhi Mu*), 5g
Radix Dioscoreae Oppositae (*Shan Yao*), 10g
Rhizoma Alismatis (*Ze Xie*), 10g
Sclerotium Poriae Cocoris (*Fu Ling*), 10
Cortex Radicis Moutan (*Dan Pi*), 10g

External treatment

Decoct a suitable amount of Rhizoma Coptidis Chinensis (*Huang Lian*) and soak the penis in this.

Yin jing duan xiao
Short penis

Abnormal shortness of the penis may result in an abnormal sex-life which is detrimental to both the physical and emotional health of the male. Although some may not consider this a disease category, TCM does offer treatment for this condition.

Bing yin bing ji
Disease causes, disease mechanisms

According to TCM theory, penile shortness is due to congenital insufficiency of the kidneys as well as damage to the liver and kidneys resulting in malnourishment of the penis, remembering that the genitalia are ruled by the kidneys and the penis is the gathering of the hundred sinews ruled by the liver.

Bian zheng lun zhi
Treatment based on pattern discrimination

1. *Yuan yin xu shang yuan yang*
Vacuity of original yin injures original yang

Pathognomic manifestations: Dizziness, poor memory, insomnia, easily awakened, palpitations, abnormal perspiration, aversion to cold, heat in the center of the palms and soles, weakness of the low back and knees, possible spermatorrhea, a short penis, and difficulty maintaining an erection, a cold sensation in the penis, scrotal tightness, a feeling of fullness and hardness in the lower abdomen, a pale tongue, and a deep, thready, slow pulse

Therapeutic principles: Supplement the kidneys, nourish the liver, and assist yang

Guiding formula:

Radix Coquitus Rehmanniae (Shu Di), 24g
Radix Dioscoreae Oppositae (*Shan Yao*), 12g
Fructus Lycii Chinensis (*Gou Qi Zi*), 12g
Herba Cistanchis (*Rou Cong Rong*), 12g
Fructus Psoraleae Corylifoliae (*Bu Gu Zhi*), 12g
Herba Epimedii (*Yin Yang Huo*), 12g
Cortex Cinnamomi (*Rou Gui*), 4.5g
Rhizoma Anemarrhenae (*Zhi Mu*), 4.5g
Radix Praeparatus Aconiti Carmichaeli (*Fu Zi*), 9g
Colla Cornu Cervi (*Lu Jiao*), 9g
Fructus Rosae Laevigatae (*Jin Ying Zi*), 15g

Yang suo
Penile retraction

Penile retraction is referred to as *yang suo* or *yin suo*. It may be either an acute or chronic condition. However, no matter if acute or chronic, severe pain always accompanies this condition. This condition is most often seen in children.

Bing yin bing ji
Disease causes, disease mechanisms

Yang suo is related to the liver and kidneys. The liver channel traverses the region of the genitalia and the kidneys rule the *er yin* or two yin, *i.e.*, the genital orifices and anus. There are three basic causes of penile retraction according to TCM. The first is cold stasis in the liver channel. This typically occurs in patients who are constitutionally yin to begin with. This then allows evil cold to invade the *jue yin* channel causing the sinews to contract and thus the penis.

The second cause of penile retraction is kidney yang vacuity. If kidney yang vacuity is coupled by cold injury, this may also result in penile retraction.

And the third cause of penile retraction is related to the stagnation of hot evils. This is a relatively rare occurrence and affects people with a yang constitution. Replete evil heat or damp heat pouring down may obstruct the flow of qi and blood to the penis. Thus the penis fails to be nourished and retracts as a species of atony.

Bian zheng lun zhi
Treatment based on pattern discrimination

1. *Gan jing han yu*
Liver channel cold stasis

Pathognomic manifestations: Lower abdominal coldness, pain, and spasm, cold extremities, penile retraction with a cold scrotum, a pale tongue with a white coating, and a thready, wiry pulse

Therapeutic principles: Warm the liver and relax the sinews

Guiding formulas:

Si Ni Tang (see above) plus *Wu Zhu Yu Tang*

Fructus Evodiae Rutecarpae (*Wu Zhu Yu*)

Radix Panacis Ginseng (*Ren Shen*)
Rhizoma Recens Zingiberis (*Sheng Jiang*)
Fructus Zizyphi Jujubae (*Da Zao*)

Nuan Gan Jian (see above) plus **Er Chen Tang** (see above)

Dang Gui Si Ni Tang

Radix Angelicae Sinensis (*Dang Gui*)
Ramulus Cinnamomi (*Gui Zhi*)
Radix Albus Paeoniae Lactiflorae (*Bai Shao*)
Herba Cum Radice Asari Seiboldi (*Xi Xin*)
Caulis Akebiae Mutong (*Mu Tong*)
Radix Praeparatus Glycyrrhizae (*Zhi Gan Cao*)
Fructus Zizyphi Jujubae (*Da Zao*)

In severe cases, use

Shao Fu Zhu Yu Tang (see above)

2. Shen gan xu han
   Kidney/liver vacuity cold

Pathognomic manifestations: Penile and scrotal retraction with chilling of the four limbs, coldness and pain of the low back and lumbar region, cold pain of the external genitalia, possible impotence, a pale face, clear, profuse urine, a pale tongue with a thin, white coating, and a sodden, slow pulse

Therapeutic principles: Supplement the liver & kidneys, warm the yang

Guiding formulas:

Shen Qi Wan a.k.a. **Ba Wei Di Huang Wan** (see above)

You Gui Wan (see above)

Shi Quan Da Bu Tang

Radix Astragali Seu Hedysari (*Huang Qi*)
Cortex Cinnamomi (*Rou Gui*)
Radix Panacis Ginseng (*Ren Shen*)
Radix Coquitus Rehmanniae (*Shu Di*)
Rhizoma Atractylodis Macrocephalae (*Bai Zhu*)
Radix Angelicae Sinensis (*Dang Gui*)
Radix Albus Paeoniae Lactiflorae (*Bai Shao*)
Rhizoma Ligustici Wallichii (*Chuan Xiong*)
Sclerotium Poriae Cocoris (*Fu Ling*)
Radix Praeparatus Glycyrrhizae (*Zhi Gan Cao*)

Shen Fu Tang

Radix Panacis Ginseng (*Ren Shen*)
Radix Praeparatus Aconiti Carmichaeli (*Fu Zi*)

3. Shang han ni qi
Cold injury, counterflow qi

Pathognomic manifestations: Coldness and pain of the external genitalia with penile retraction, tightness and congestion in the lower abdomen and chest, moodiness changing from depression to anger to frustration, a pale tongue with a white coating, and a slow or wiry pulse

Therapeutic principles: Warm and descend counterflow qi

Guiding formula:

Flos Caryophylli (*Ding Xiang*), 1-3g
Fructus Evodiae Rutecarpae (*Wu Zhu Yu*), 2-6g
Fructus Meliae Toosendanis (*Chuan Lian Zi*), 12-24g
Semen Litchi Chinensis (*Li Zhi He*), 15-20g
Radix Praeparatus Glycyrrhizae (*Zhi Gan Cao*), 5g

4. *Shi re xia zhu*
Damp heat pouring downward

Pathognomic manifestations: Penile retraction with dryness of the throat and mouth, spasm and pain of the lower abdomen, painful, difficult urination, a red tongue with a yellow coating, and a rapid pulse

Therapeutic principles: Discharge fire and relax the sinews

Guiding formulas:

Long Dan Xie Gan Tang (see above)

San Ren Tang (see above)

Acupuncture/moxibustion therapy

Acupuncture treatments

1. *Guan Yuan* (CV 4) and *Chang Qiang* (GV 1); strong stimulation

2. *Hui Yin* (CV 1), *Zhong Ji* (CV 3), and *Guan Yuan* (CV 4); strong stimulation

3. *Ren Zhong* (GV 26), *Bai Hui* (GV 20), *Ming Men* (GV 4), *Yao Yang Guang* (GV 3), *Wei Zhong* (Bl 40), *Wei Yang* (Bl 39), *Zu San Li* (St 36), and *San Yin Jiao* (Sp 6)

Moxibustion treatment

Moxa directly on *San Yin Jiao* (Sp 6), *Qi Hai* (CV 6), *Guan Yuan* (CV 4), and *Bai Hui* (GV 20). Moxa the penis itself indirectly.

Acupuncture & moxibustion

Needle *Guan Yuan* (CV 4), *Shen Shu* (Bl 23), *San Yin Jiao* (Sp 6), and *Nei Guan* (Per 6); then moxa *Guan Yuan* and *Shen Shu*.

Electro-acupuncture

Qi Hai (CV 6), *Guan Yuan* (CV 4), *Li Gou* (Liv 5), and *Tai Chong* (Liv 3)

恬淡虚無，真氣
從之，精神内守，
病安從来。
"素問・上古天真論"

Emotions cannot be seen, but the true qi follows them;
if the spirit is kept inside, how can one become diseased?

4

Yin Nan Bing Scrotal Diseases

Yin nan shi zheng
Damp scrotal sores

Damp scrotal sores are characterized by dryness and itching in the scrotal area which turn into ulceration and oozing of pus after scratching.

Bing yin bing ji
Disease causes, disease mechanisms

Damp scrotal sores are primarily due to damp heat invading the scrotal area.

Bian zheng lun zhi
Treatment based on pattern discrimination

1. *Shi re gong xia*
Damp heat attacks below

Pathognomic manifestations: Dryness and itching of the scrotum follwed by ulceration and oozing of pus after scratching

Therapeutic principles: Clear heat and disinhibit dampness, dispel wind and stop itching

Guiding formula: *Long Dan Xie Gan Tang* (see above) plus medicinals to dispel wind and stop itching, such as:

Radix Sophorae Flavescentis (*Ku Shen*)
Semen Cnidii Monnieri (*She Chuan Zi*)
Cortex Fructi Benincasae Hispidae (*Dong Gua Pi*)
Rhizoma Dioscoreae Hypoglaucae (*Bi Xie*)
Fructus Kochiae Scopariae (*Di Fu Zi*)

External treatment

Grind equal portions of the following medicinals into a fine
powder and mix with petroleum jelly to form a paste:

Pulvis Indigonis (*Qing Dai*)
Lithargyrum (*Mi Tuo Shen*)
Sulphur (*Liu Huang*)
Talcum (*Hua Shi*)

One may also fumigate and wash with:

Folium Artemesiae Argyii (*Ai Ye*), 30g
Herba Senecionis (*Qian Li Guang*), 30g

Decoct in water for 15 minutes. Wash the affected area 1 time per
day, with 10 times comprising 1 course of treatment.

One may wash with, and/or drink the following decoction:

Semen Cnidii Monnieri (*She Chuang Zi*), 15g
Cortex Phellodendri (*Huang Bai*), 30g
Radix Sophorae Flavescentis (*Ku Shen*), 60g
Flos Lonicerae Japonicae (*Yin Hua*), 30g

Acupuncture/moxibustion therapy

Acupuncture treatment

Needle *San Yin Jiao* (Sp 6), *Xue Hai* (Sp 10), *Zu San Li* (St 36), and *Qu Chi* (LI 11).

Moxibustion treatment

Indirectly moxa the entire scrotal area.

Yin nan sheng lou
Scrotal leaking & discharge

Scrotal leaking and discharge refers to scrotal lesions which exude a milky fluid. This condition is not commonly encountered in clinical practice.

Bing yin bing ji
Disease causes, disease mechanisms

TCM regards scrotal leaking and discharge as either the result of kidney vacuity not consolidating body fluids or damp heat accumulating in the lower burner. Kidney vacuity may be due to any of a number of causes including age, chronic disease, congenital weakness, taxation of various sorts, etc. The causes of damp heat accumulating in the lower burner and genitalia have been described above.

Bian zheng lun zhi
Treatment based on pattern discrimination

1. *Shen qi bu gu*
Kidney qi not consolidating

Pathognomic manifestations: Milky discharge, lower abdominal distention, stuffy chest, difficult urination, low back and knee soreness and weakness, possible spermatorrhea or premature ejaculation, a pale tongue, and a sodden, slow, or slippery pulse

Therapeutic principles: Warm the kidneys and astringe body fluids

Guiding formula: *Jin Gui Shen Qi Wan* a.k.a. *Ba Wei Di Huang Wan* (see above) plus:

Os Calcinatus Draconis (*Duan Long Gu*)
Concha Calcinata Ostreae (*Duan Mu Li*)
Herba Epimedii (*Yin Yang Huo*)
Fructus Lycii Chinensis (*Gou Qi Zi*)

2. *Shi re xia zhu*
Damp heat pouring down

Pathognomic manifestations: Turbid, milky discharge with a hot, painful feeling on urination, a dry mouth, thirst, a red tongue with slimy, yellow coating, and a slippery, rapid pulse

Therapeutic principles: Clear heat and disinhibit dampness

Guiding formulas:

Long Dan Xie Gan Tang (see above)

Bi Xie Fen Qing Yin (see above)

Yin nan wei suo
Scrotal atony & retraction

This pathocondition is a species of *wei zheng* or atonic condition. It is due to the shrinking and contraction of the scrotal muscles.

Bing yin bing ji
Disease causes, disease mechanisms

TCM regards this condition as the result of qi stagnation and blood stasis causing a failure in the qi and blood's nourishing the scrotum. Qi stagnation is mostly due to emotional frustration, with blood stasis the eventual end result of such stagnation, if that stagnation is pronounced or prolonged.

Bian zheng lun zhi
Treatment based on pattern discrimination

1. Qi zhi xue yu
Qi stagnation, blood stasis

Pathognomic manifestations: Persistent scrotal retraction, possible palpitations, red face, dream-disturbed sleep, headache, dry mouth, a purple tongue, and a thready, astringent/grating pulse

Therapeutic principles: Move and regulate the qi, activate the blood and transform stasis

Guiding formula: *Xue Fu Zhu Yu Tang* (see above) plus

Semen Allii Tuberosi (*Jiu Cai Zi*)
Semen Cnidii Monnieri (*She Chuang Zi*)

Yin nan xue guang liu
Scrotal blood vessel tumor

This condition refers to hemangioma of the scrotum. It consists of increased vascularization of a localized region of the scrotum and is accompanied by itching. If scratched, blood may appear. This condition is rarely seen and resembles *xue zhi* or bloody mole.

Bing yin bing ji
Disease causes, disease mechanisms

This condition is due to stagnant fire damaging the channels resulting from yin vacuity. The causes of yin vacuity have been discussed above.

Bian zheng lun zhi
Treatment based on pattern discrimination

1. Yu huo shang jing
Stagnant fire injuring the channels

Pathognomic manifestations: Increased local vascularization in the scrotum, itching, possible bleeding after scratching, heat in the five centers, dry mouth but no desire to drink, possible dizziness and tinnitus, low back and knee soreness and weakness, a red tongue with scant coating, and a thready, rapid pulse

Therapeutic principles: Enrich yin and clear heat, stop bleeding

Guiding formula:

Plastrum Praeparatum Testudinis (*Zhi Gui Ban*) 12g
Fructus Ligustri Lucidi (*Nu Zhen Zi*), 10g
Herba Ecliptae Prostratae (*Han Lian Cao*), 10g
Fructus Gardeniae Jasminoidis (*Shan Zhi Zi*), 10g
Radix Carbonisatus Sanguisorbae (*Di Yu Tan*), 10g

Cortex Phellodendri (*Chuan Huang Bai*), 5g
Radix Carbonisatus Rubiae Cordifoliae (*Qian Cao Tan*), 6g
Radix Albus Paeoniae Lactiflorae (*Bai Shao*), 6g
Radix Rehmanniae (*Sheng Di Huang*), 15g

Yin nan du a.k.a. *Yin nan huai zhu*
Scrotal toxins

This condition resembles acute inflammation of the scrotum in that the scrotal skin is red and swollen. The onset of this condition is rapid and, if treatment is delayed, the scrotal skin may be sloughed off, exposing the testes underneath.

Bing yin bing ji
Disease causes, disease mechanisms

According to TCM, the cause of scrotal toxicity is a combination of righteous qi insufficiency and liver channel damp heat pouring downward. The causes of damp heat in the liver channel have been described above.

Bian zheng lun zhi
Treatment based on pattern discrimination

1. *Gan jing shi re xia zhu*
Liver channel damp heat pouring downward

Pathognomic manifestations: Itchy, red, painful, swollen scrotum, possible fever, dry mouth, red eyes, insomnia, a red tongue with white coating, and a wiry, slippery pulse

Therapeutic principles: Clear and disinhibit liver channel dampness and heat, discharge liver fire and resolve toxins

Guiding formula: *Long Dan Xie Gan Tang Jia Jian*

Radix Gentianae Scabrae (*Long Dan Cao*), 5g
Caulis Akebiae Mutong (*Mu Tong*), 5g
Radix Bupleuri (*Chai Hu*), 5g
Radix Scutellariae Baicalensis (*Huang Qin*), 6g
Rhizoma Alismatis (*Ze Xie*), 10g
Semen Plantaginis (*Che Qian Zi*), 10g
Radix Angelicae Sinensis (*Dang Gui*), 10g
Fructus Forsythiae Suspensae (*Lian Qiao*), 10g
Radix Rehmanniae (*Sheng Di*), 12g
Radix Glycyrrhizae (*Gan Cao*), 3g
Rhizoma Coptidis Chinensis (*Huang Lian*), 3g

Zi yong
Testicular *yong*

Yong is a general term for acute, localized, suppurative inflammatory lesions of the skin and subcutaneous tissues, or of the five viscera. Purulent ulceration of the scrotum with redness, swelling, local heat, and pain are referred to in Chinese medicine as testicular *yong*. If not treated in time, testicular *yong* may be accompanied by such generalized symptoms as fever, aversion to cold, dry mouth, thirst with a desire for hot drinks, yellow urine, and other such complications. In severe cases, excessive pus formation in the local area can be seen.

Bing yin bing ji
Disease causes, disease mechanisms

This condition is due to deep pentration of damp heat into the muscles and sinews, thus creating stasis within the channels and connecting vessels.

Bian zheng lun zhi
Treatment based on pattern discrimination

1. *Shi re jia yu zuo jing luo*
Damp heat (causing) binding stasis
in the channels & connecting vessels

Pathognomic manifestations: Purulent ulceration of the srotum with redness, localized heat, swelling, and pain, possible exudation of excessive pus, possible fever and aversion to chill, dry mouth and thirst, yellow urine, dry stools, a red tongue with a yellow coating, and a thready, wiry, rapid pulse

Therapeutic principles: Clear and disinhibit dampness and heat, harmonize the qi and blood and resolve toxins

Guiding formula:

Fructus Meliae Toosendanis (*Chuan Lian Zi*), 6g
Rhizoma Alismatis (*Ze Xie*), 6g
Fructus Forsythiae Suspensae (*Lian Qiao*), 6g
Herba Cum Radice Lobeliae Chinensis (*Ban Bian Lian*), 6g
Pericarpium Citri Reticulatae (*Qing Pi*),3g
Radix Glycyrrhizae (*Gan Cao*), 3g
Radix Rubrus Paeoniae Lactiflorae (*Chi Shao*), 4.5g
Herba Cum Radice Violae Yedoensis (*Zi Hua Di Ding*), 15g

The diagnosis and treatment of testicular *yong* can also be divided into acute and chronic inflammatory stages. The chronic stage may develop from the acute stage or one may develop chronic testicular *yong* without passing through a manifest acute stage. In chronic testicular *yong* there is usually a gradual increase in cruelly persistent pain. Chronic testicular *yong* is often quite complicated and typically involves affections of the liver, kidney, heart, and spleen channels due to a combination of damp heat, toxins, phlegm, and stasis. Therefore, there are a number of different treatment methods which may be applied, depending upon the individual patient's signs and symptoms and disease mechanisms.

If toxins are prominent, one can resolve toxins by using:

Radix Et Rhizoma Rhei (*Da Huang*)
Radix Praeparatus Aconiti Carmichaeli (*Fu Zi*)
Herba Oldenlandiae Diffusae (*Bai Hua She She Cao*)
Fructus Meliae Toosendanis (*Chuan Lian Zi*)
Semen Citri (*Ju He*)
Radix Rubrus Paeoniae Lactiflorae (*Chi Shao*)

In this formula, Radix Praeparatus Aconiti Carmichaeli and Radix Et Rhizoma Rhei are used together, based on the fact that, although there is fever and heat, there is also fear of chill and, therefore, cold. The key to their successful use together is their respective correct dosages.

If dampness and heat are prominent, then one should clear heat and disinhibit dampness using **Long Dan Xie Gan Tang** (see above) plus:

Fructus Meliae Toosendanis (*Chuan Lian Zi*)
Semen Litchi Chinensis (*Li Zhi He*)
Semen Citri (*Ju He*)
Herba Cum Radice Taraxaci Mongolici (*Pu Gong Ying*)
Spicae Prunellae Vulgaris (*Xia Gu Cao*)

In order to dispel stasis through the urine and feces, one can use **Huang Lian Jie Du Tang Jia Wei.**

Rhizoma Coptidis Chinensis (*Huang Lian*)
Radix Scutellariae Baicalensis (*Huang Qin*)
Cortex Phellodendri (*Huang Bai*)
Fructus Gardeniae Jasminoidis (*Shan Zhi Zi*)
Radix Et Rhizoma Rhei (*Da Huang*)
Mirabilitum (*Xuan Ming Fen*)
Folium Sennae (*Fan Xie Ye*)

Sclerotium Poriae Cocoris (*Fu Ling*)
Rhizoma Alismatis (*Ze Xie*)
Semen Plantaginis (*Che Qian Zi*)

In order to clear heat from the *ying* and *xue*, one can use **Qing Ying Tang Jia Wei**

Cornu Rhinoceri (*Xi Jiao*)
Radix Rehmanniae (*Sheng Di*)
Radix Scrophulariae Ningpoensis (*Yuan Shen*)
Tuber Ophiopogonis Japonicae (*Mai Dong*)
Herba Lophatheri Gracilis (*Zhu Ye*)
Rhizoma Coptidis Chinensis (*Huang Lian*)
Flos Lonicerae Japonicae (*Yin Hua*)
Fructus Forsythiae Suspensae (*Lian Qiao*)
Radix Salviae Miltiorrhizae (*Dan Shen*)
Radix Isatidis Seu Baphacacanthi (*Ban Lan Geng*)

In order to transform phlegm and soften hardness, one can use **Xiao Jin Dan**

Resina Liquidambaris Taiwanianae (*Bai Jiao Xiang*)
Radix Aconiti (*Cao Wu*)
Feces Trogopterori Seu Pteromi (*Wu Ling Zhi*)
Lumbricus (*Di Long*)
Semen Momordicae Cochinensis (*Mu Bie*)
Gummum Olibani (*Ru Xiang*)
Myrrha (*Mo Yao*)
Radix Angelicae Sinensis (*Dang Gui Shen*)
Secretio Moschi Moschiferi (*She Xiang*)
Carbonized inkstick (*Mo Tan*)

In order to regulate the qi and resolve toxins, one can use:

Fructus Meliae Toosendanis (*Chuan Lian Zi*)
Radix Linderae Strychnifoliae (*Tai Wu Yao*)
Radix Saussureae Seu Vladimiriae (*Mu Xiang*)

Radix Astragali Seu Hedysari (*Huang Qi*)
Rhizoma Atractylodis Macrocephalae (*Bai Zhu*)
Radix Codonopsis Pilosulae (*Dang Shen*)
Radix Salviae Miltiorrhizae (*Dan Shen*)
Semen Pruni Persicae (*Tao Ren*)
Semen Coicis Lachryma-jobi (*Yi Yi Ren*)
Herba Lycopi Lucidi (*Ze Lan*)

In order to activate the blood and clear turbidity, one can use:

Radix Salviae Miltiorrhizae (*Dan Shen*)
Cortex Radicis Moutan (*Dan Pi*)
Rhizoma Sparganii (*San Leng*)
Rhizoma Curcumae Zedoariae (*E Zhu*)
Semen Pruni Persicae (*Tao Ren*)
Semen Coicis Lachryma-jobi (*Yi Yi Ren*)
Herba Cum Radice Taraxaci Mongolici (*Pu Gong Ying*)
Cortex Phellodendri (*Huang Bai*)
Rhizoma Dioscoreae Hypoglaucae (*Bi Xie*)
Rhizoma Smilacis Glabrae (*Tu Fu Ling*)
Talcum (*Hua Shi*)
Radix Glycyrrhizae (*Gan Cao*)

In order to nourish water and enrich the kidneys, one can use **Zhi Bai Di Huang Wan** (see above).

In order to warm the channels and transform stasis, one can use:

Fructus Piperi Longis (*Bi Ba*)
Semen Citri (*Ju He*)
Rhizoma Alpiniae Officinari (*Gao Liang Jiang*)
Rhizoma Corydalis Yanhusuo (*Yuan Hu*)
Caulis Akebiae Mutong (*Mu Tong*)
Fructus Foeniculi Vulgaris (*Xiao Hui Xiang*)
Fructus Meliae Toosendanis (*Chuan Lian Zi*)

Acupuncture/moxibustion therapy

One can needle and/or moxa from among the following points:

Da Dun (Liv 1), *Tai Chong* (Liv 3), *Zhong Fen* (Liv 4), *Qu Quan* (Liv 8), *Guan Yuan* (CV 4), *Qi Hai* (CV 6), *Gui Lai* (St 29), *San Yin Jiao* (Sp 6), and *He Gu* (LI 4)

Zi tong
Testicular pain

Testicular pain is also called in Chinese *shen zi tong* or kidney egg pain. In terms of modern Western medicine, it is usually due to chronic prostatitis, trauma, variocele, spermatocystitis, seminal cysts, hydrocele, and other such conditions and complications.

Bing yin bing ji
Disease causes, disease mechanisms

According to TCM, there is no pain if there is free flow and, if there is not free flow, there is pain. Therefore, all patterns pertaining to testicular pain have at their root, obstruction to the free and patent flow of qi and blood to and through the testes. The first cause of testicular pain is due to cold and damp evils accumulating in the liver channel. This obstructs the free flow of qi and blood resulting in stasis, swelling, and pain. The second cause of testicular pain is damp heat pouring down and obstructing the free flow of qi and blood. The causes of damp heat have been discussed above. The third cause is depressive heat in the liver channel. This likewise obstructs the free and patent flow of qi and blood in the area of the genitals. And the fourth mechanism causing testicular pain is liver/kidney yin vacuity. In this case, it is actually liver heat which causes the pain. However, because this heat also injures and damages the blood and *jing*, the patient also displays signs and symptoms of liver blood and kidney yin vacuity.

Bian zheng lun zhi
Treatment based on pattern discrimination

1. Han shi nei qin
Cold dampness intrude internally

Pathognomic manifestations: Rapid disease onset, swelling and pain of the testes and a dragging or falling feeling, swelling of the scrotal skin, aversion to cold, lower abdominal pain, resists pressure, a thick, white tongue coating, and a deep, wiry pulse

Therapeutic principles: Warm and scatter cold and dampness, course the liver and stop pain

Guiding formulas:

Ju Ju Tang Jia Jian

Fructus Citri Reticulatae (*Ju Ju*), 10g
Fructus Meliae Toosendanis (*Chuan Lian Zi*), 10g
Radix Gentianae Macrocephyllae (*Qin Jiao*), 10g
Radix Ledebouriellae Sesloidis (*Fang Feng*), 10g
Rhizoma Alismatis (*Ze Xie*), 10g
Radix Rubrus Paeoniae Lactiflorae (*Chi Shao*), 10g
Radix Praeparatus Glycyrrhizae (*Zhi Gan Cao*), 10g
Fructus Foeniculi Vulgaris (*Xiao Hui Xiang*), 10g
Rhizoma Alpiniae Officinari (*Gao Liang Jiang*), 10g
Semen Citri (*Ju He*), 15g
Semen Litchi Chinensis (*Li Zhi He*), 15g
Rhizoma Corydalis Yanhusuo (*Yuan Hu*), 15g

Dang Gui Si Ni Tang (see above) plus Ju He Wan

Semen Citri (*Ju He*)
Fructus Meliae Toosendanis (*Chuan Lian Zi*)
Rhizoma Corydalis Yanhusuo (*Yuan Hu*)
Cortex Magnoliae Officinalis (*Hou Po*)

Fructus Immaturus Citri Seu Ponciri (*Zhi Shi*)
Cortex Cinnamomi (*Rou Gui*)
Thallus Algae (*Kun Bu*)
Herba Sargassi (*Hai Zao*)
Herba Laminariae Japonicae (*Hai Dai*)
Semen Pruni Persicae (*Tao Ren*)
Caulis Akebiae Mutong (*Mu Tong*)
Radix Saussureae Seu Vladimiriae (*Mu Xiang*)

2. *Shi re xia zhu*
Damp heat pouring down

Pathognomic manifestations: Testicular swelling, enlargement, and pain, scrotum red and swollen, movement not easy, fever, heart vexation, chest and flank distention and oppression, a dry, bitter mouth, yellow/red urination, dry stools, a thick, slimy tongue coating, and a sodden, rapid pulse

Therapeutic principles: Clear heat and eliminate dampness, course the liver and resolve toxins

Guiding formulas:

Long Dan Xie Gan Tang (see above)

Gan Lu Xiao Du Dan Jia Jian

Cortex Radicis Moutan (*Dan Pi*), 150g
Fructus Gardeniae Jasminoidis (*Zhi Zi*), 150g
Fructus Forsythiae Suspensae (*Lian Qiao*), 150g
Herba Artemesiae Capillaris (*Yin Chen*), 200g
Talcum (*Hua Shi*), 450g
Radix Bupleuri (*Chai Hu*), 120g
Radix Scutellariae Baicalensis (*Huang Qin*), 120g
Radix Sophorae Flavescentis (*Ku Shen*), 120g
Rhizoma Alismatis (*Ze Xie*), 120g
Caulis Akebiae Mutong (*Mu Tong*), 200g

Grind into powder. Each time take 9g. Or, one may reduce the amounts of each ingredient and decoct in water and take.

3. Gan jing yu re
Liver channel depressive heat

Pathognomic manifestations: Swelling and enlargement of the testes, heat, aching, and *yong* associated with lower abdominal pain, scrotal redness and swelling, fever, fear of cold, urination short and red, dizziness and tinnitus, vexation and stuffiness within the heart, a yellow tongue coating, and a wiry, rapid pulse

Therapeutic principles: Clear the heat and course the liver, activate the blood and disperse stasis

Guiding formula: *Long Dan Xie Gan Tang* (see above) plus:

Rhizoma Ligustici Wallichii (*Chuan Xiong*)
Radix Angelicae (*Bai Zhi*)
Gummum Olibani (*Ru Xiang*)
Myrrha (*Mo Yao*)

4. Gan shen yin xu
Liver/kidney yin vacuity

Pathognomic manifestations: Enlargement and swelling of the testes, scrotal dampness, swelling, and pain, vertigo and dizziness, soreness and weakness of the low back and knees, vexatious heat in the five centers, a red tongue with scant coating, and a deep, thready, rapid pulse. This mostly occurs in adolescents.

Therapeutic principles: Enrich yin and nourish the kidneys, disperse swelling and stop pain

Guiding formula: *Liu Wei Di Huang Wan Jia Wei*

Radix Rehmanniae (*Sheng Di*)

Fructus Corni Officinalis (*Shan Zhu Yu*)
Radix Dioscoreae Oppositae (*Shan Yao*)
Cortex Radicis Moutan (*Dan Pi*)
Sclerotium Poriae Cocoris (*Fu Ling*)
Fructus Lycii Chinensis (*Gou Qi*)
Rhizoma Corydalis Yanhusuo (*Yuan Hu*)
Fructus Meliae Toosendanis (*Jin Ling Zi*)
Semen Litchi Chinensis (*Li Zhi He*)

External treatment

Cortex Radicis Kadsurae (*Zi Jing Pi*), 150g
Radix Angelicae Pubescentis (*Du Huo*), 90g
Radix Rubrus Paeoniae Lactiflorae (*Chi Shao*), 60g
Radix Angelicae (*Bai Zhi*), 30g
Rhizoma Acori Graminei (*Shi Chang Pu*), 45g

Grind into a fine powder, then mix with either onion juice or aged wine and apply to the affected area.

Sai xian yan xing gao huan yan
Scrotal inflammation due to mumps

This condition is a complication of mumps. Its signs and symptoms are swelling and pain, redness and heat of the scrotum in a person already suffering from mumps. It is most commonly met with amongst children. In adult males, this condition may result in sterility.

Bing yin bing ji
Disease causes, disease mechanisms

Mumps is caused by invasion of wind heat evils which block the *shao yang*. Because the *shao yang* and *jue yin* are connected, this evil heat may enter the *jue yin* causing blockage at the level of the genitalia with swelling, redness, heat, and pain.

Bian zheng lun zhi
Treatment based on pattern discrimination

1. Jue yin re du
Hot toxins in the jue yin

Pathognomic manifestations: Swelling, redness, inflammation, and pain of the scrotum and testes in a person already suffering from mumps, a yellow tongue coating, and a flooding, rapid pulse

Therapeutic principles: Clear heat and resolve toxins, disperse swelling and stop pain

Guiding formulas:

Xiao Chai Hu Tang He Shi Zao Tang Jia Wei

Radix Bupleuri (*Chai Hu*)
Radix Scutellariae Baicalensis (*Huang Qin*)
Radix Codonopsis Pilosulae (*Dang Shen*)
Rhizoma Pinelliae Ternatae (*Ban Xia*)
Fructus Zizyphi Jujubae (*Da Zao*)
Radix Praeparatus Glycyrrhizae (*Zhi Gan Cao*)
Rhizoma Recens Zingiberis (*Sheng Jiang*)
Radix Euphorbiae Kansui (*Gan Sui*)
Radix Euphorbiae Seu Knoxiae (*Jing Da Ji*)
Flos Daphnis Genkwae (*Yuan Hua*)
Herba Sargassi (*Hai Zao*)
Semen Citri (*Ju He*)
Radix Isatidis Seu Baphicacanthi (*Ban Lang Geng*)

Unnamed formula

Spica Prunellae Vulgaris (*Xia Gu Cao*)
Radix Bupleuri (*Chai Hu*)

Rhizoma Corydalis Yanhusuo (*Yuan Hu*)
Fructus Meliae Toosendanis (*Chuan Lian Zi*)
Rhizoma Sparganii (*San Leng*)
Rhizma Curcumae Zedoariae (*E Zhu*)
Semen Pruni Persicae (*Tao Ren*)
Semen Litchi Chinensis (*Li Zhi He*)

External treatment

Pulvis Indigonis (*Qing Dai*), 1.5g
Borneolum (*Bing Pian*), 1.5g
Realgar (*Xiong Huang*), 5g
Alum (*Ming Fan*), 3g

Grind into powder and mix with petroleum jelly to form a paste. Apply to the affected area, cover and hold in place with gauze.

Shan qi
Hernias

Shan qi refers to a group of pathoconditons which all manifest in the inguinal, scrotal regions, and lower abdominal regions. Most premodern TCM texts speak of a number of various types of *shan*. Since only some of these are actually species of hernia according to modern Western medicine, the term *shan* presents special difficulty to the translator. The most common types of *shan* in the traditional literature include the *hu shan* (foxlike *shan*), *han shan* (cold *shan*), *shui shan* (water *shan*), *qi shan* (umbilical *shan*), *tui shan* referring to swelling, pain, hardening, or numbness of the scrotum, *tui shan* also referring to testicular hardness, swelling, dragging pain, and/or numbness, *qi shan*, *xue shan* (bloody *shan*), *jin shan* (sinew, *i.e.*, penile *shan*), and *pan shan* (disk *shan*). Since some of these have been discussed under the category of *zi tong*, testicular pain, we will only discuss *hu shan* (foxlike *shan*), and *shui shan* (water *shan*), below.

A. *Hu shan*
Foxlike *shan*

Similar to *qi shan* which is swelling and pain on one side of the scrotum radiating to the lumbar region, *hu shan* is when a part of the small intestine intermittently descends into the scrotum. This occurs only when the patient stands up and disappears when the patient lies down. It is called foxlike *shan* since this appearance and disappearance is like a fox darting in and out of its den. It is most commonly seen in the elderly, children, and/or weak and debilitated patients. This Chinese disease category essentially is identical to inguino-femoral hernia in modern Western medicine.

Bing yin bing ji
Disease causes, disease mechanisms

According to TCM theory, foxlike *shan* is due to spleen/kidney insufficiency failing to lift, restrain, and consolidate the abdominal contents. This may be due to congenital weakness, aging, chronic sickness and debility, or any other factor resulting in deficiency and weakness of these two organs. In addition, foxlike *shan* may also be due to cold damp stagnation. Typically this occurs as a result of spleen/kidney vacuity failing to promote the transportation and transformation of body fluids. In Chinese medicine, it is said that the liver channel traverses the sides of the abdomen. If dampness and cold fall down into this area of the lower abdomen, the liver channel loses its ability to course and discharge, and thus intermittent swellings in this region occur.

Bian zheng lun zhi
Treatment based on pattern discrimination

1. *Han shi zu gan jue yin*
Cold dampness obstructs the *jue yin*

Pathognomic manifestations: Scrotal swelling, pain with a dragging feeling in the scrotum, pain radiating to the lower abdomen, pain aggravated by cough, swelling appears when standing and disappears when lying down

Therapeutic principles: Disinhibit dampness and warm the channels, soothe liver qi and strengthen the spleen

Guiding formulas:

Xian Hui He Ji

Herba Agrimoniae Pilosae (*Xian He Cao*), 9-15g
Fructus Foeniculi Vulgaris (*Xiao Hui Xiang*), 2-3g
Rhizoma Recens Zingiberis (*Sheng Jiang*), 1-2g
Rice wine (*Mi Jiu*), 20-80ml

Unnamed formula

Fructus Meliae Toosendanis (*Chuan Lian Zi*)
Fructus Foeniculi Vulgaris (*Xiao Hui Xiang*)
Herba Epimedii (*Yin Yang Huo*)
Semen Trigonellae Foeni-greaci (*Hu Lu Ba*)
Sclerotium Poriae Cocoris (*Fu Ling*)
Rhizoma Pinelliae Ternatae (*Ban Xia*)
Cortex Eucommiae Ulmoidis (*Du Zhong*)
Semen Allii Tuberosi (*Jiu Zi*)
Fructus Seu Semen Amomi (*Sha Ren*)
Radix Ledebouriellae Sesloidis (*Fang Feng*)
Radix Angelicae Sinensis (*Dang Gui*)
Os Sepiae Seu Sepiellae (*Dan Yu Gu*)
Fructus Evodiae Rutecarpae (*Wu Zhu Yu*)

Grind into powder and make into pills with water. Take 2 times per day, 7.5g each time.

Acupuncture therapy

Needle *Qi Chong* (St 30), *Ti Tuo* (N-CA-4), *Zhong Ji* (CV 3), *Guan Yuan* (CV 4), and *Bai Hui* (GV 20)

Before commencing each acupuncture treatment, the patient should empty his bladder. While being treated, the patient should lie down so as to help push the hernia up and in. Treat once every other day, 12 treatments constituting 1 course.

B. *Shui shan*
Water *shan*

This traditional Chinese pathocondition is similar to hydrocele in modern Western medicine. Patients with this condition suffer from swelling of the testes on one or both sides, enlargement of the testes, and crystalization. This condition may result in other urinary and sexual dysfunction diseases. Typically, there is no inflammation, redness, or pain associated with this condition unless treatment is delayed.

Bing yin bing ji
Disease causes, disease mechanisms

The causes of this condition are similar to foxlike *shan* in that TCM mainly ascribes this condition to problems with the spleen, kidneys, and liver. Since the liver channel traverses the inguinal region, liver qi stagnation due to emotional frustration may predispose the body to attack by cold dampness in this region. If this persists, it may also become complicated by blood stasis since qi moves the blood and if the qi is obstructed, over time, the blood will become static. Secondly, if either the spleen or kidneys fail to maintain proper transformation and transportation of body fluids, dampness may be formed which, because it is heavy, may accumulate in this region. Vacuity of the spleen and/or kidneys may be either simple qi vacuity or may progress to yang vacuity. Further, if treatment is delayed, such accumulation and obstruction by evil yin may transform into damp heat. Should damp heat continue unabated, over time evil heat will injure and damage kidney yin. Since yin and qi are mutually dependent, kidney qi will not be able to transport and transform liquids, which will continue to accumulate below. However, this will be accompanied by signs and symptoms of yin vacuity above.

Bian zheng lun zhi
Treatment based on pattern discrimination

1. *Han shi zu gan jue yin*
Cold dampness obstructs the *jue yin*

Pathognomic manifestations: Swelling and enlargement of the scrotum and testes on one or both sides, chilly pain in the lower abdomen, a heavy dragging feeling in the lower abdomen, lower abdomen resists pressure but discomfort is ameliorated by warmth

Therapeutic principles: Course the liver and warm the channels, disinhibit dampness and disperse swelling

Guiding formulas:

Jia Wei Si Ling San

Sclerotium Polypori Umbellati (*Zhu Ling*), 10g
Sclerotium Poriae Cocoris (*Fu Ling*), 10g
Rhizoma Alismatis (*Ze Xie*), 10g
Semen Citri (*Ju He*), 10g
Fructus Meliae Toosendanis (*Chuan Lian Zi*), 10g
Herba Sargassi (*Hai Zao*), 10g
Cortex Cinnamomi (*Rou Gui*), 5g
Fructus Evodiae Rutecarpae (*Wu Zhu Yu*), 5g
Fructus Foeniculi Vulgaris (*Xiao Hui Xiang*), 5g
Semen Litchi Chinensis (*Li Zhi He*), 15g
Rhizoma Dioscoreae Hypoglaucae (*Bi Xie*), 15g

If accompanied by blood stasis, use *Ling Gui Zhu Gan Tang Jia Wei*

Sclerotium Poriae Cocoris (*Fu Ling*), 30g
Ramulus Cinnamomi (*Gui Zhi*), 18g
Rhizoma Atractylodis Macrocephalae (*Bai Zhu*), 18g
Thallus Algae (*Kun Bu*), 20g
Herba Sargassi (*Hai Zao*), 20g
Radix Glycyrrhizae (*Gan Cao*), 10g
Flos Carthami Tinctorii (*Hong Hua*), 10g
Semen Pruni Persicae (*Tao Ren*), 10g
Fructus Meliae Toosendanis (*Chuan Lian Zi*), 15g
Semen Litchi Chinensis (*Li He Zi*), 15g

2. *Pi qi xu*
Spleen qi vacuity

Pathognomic manifestations: Swelling of the testicles and scrotum, a dragging sensation, absence of pain, digestive complaints such as lack of appetite, abdominal distention, chest stuffiness, dizziness upon standing, fatigue, lack of strength in the extremities, and a pale tongue with thin, white coating, and a short, weak, possibly deep pulse

Therapeutic principles: Supplement the spleen and boost the qi

Guiding formula: *San He Bu Zhong Tang*

Radix Astragali Seu Hedysari (*Huang Qi*)
Radix Panacis Ginseng (*Ren Shen*)
Rhizoma Atractylodis Macrocephalae (*Bai Zhu*)
Radix Preaparatus Glycyrrhizae (*Zhi Gan Cao*)
Radix Angelicae Sinensis (*Dang Gui*)
Rhizoma Cimicifugae (*Sheng Ma*)
Radix Bupleuri (*Chai Hu*)
Pericarpium Citri Reticulatae (*Chen Pi*)
Semen Citri (*Ju He*)

Semen Litchi Chinensis (*Li Zhi He*)
Semen Mangiferae Indicae (*Mang Guo He*)
Radix Albus Paeoniae Lactiflorae (*Bai Shao*)
Semen Trigonellae Foeni-graeci (*Hu Lu Ba*)
Fructus Foeniculi Vulgaris (*Xiao Hui Xiang*)
Fructus Meliae Toosendanis (*Chuan Lian Zi*)
Sclerotium Poriae Cocoris (*Fu Ling*)

3. Yang xu
Yang vacuity

Pathognomic manifestations: Swelling of the testes and scrotum, lack of pain, edema, dysuria, dizziness, shortness of breath, palpitations below the umbilicus, low back soreness and weakness, chilled lower extremities, a pale tongue with a white, slimy coating, and a deep, weak pulse

Therapeutic principles: Warm yang and disinhibit water, disperse swelling and soften the hard

Guiding formulas:

Wu Ling San Jia Wei

Rhizoma Alismatis (*Ze Xie*)
Sclerotium Poriae Cocoris (*Fu Ling*)
Sclerotium Polypori Umbellati (*Zhu Ling*)
Ramulus Cinnamomi (*Gui Zhi*)
Rhizoma Atractylodis Macrocephalae (*Bai Zhu*)
Radix Praeparatus Aconiti Carmichaeli (*Fu Zi*)
Semen Citri (*Ju He*)
Semen Litchi Chinensis (*Li Zhi He*)
Fructus Foeniculi Vulgaris (*Xiao Hui Xiang*)
Herba Sargassi (*Hai Zao*)
Thallus Algae (*Kun Bu*)

Unnamed formula:

Radix Coquitus Rehmanniae (*Shu Di*), 5g
Sclerotium Poriae Cocoris (*Fu Ling*), 15g
Radix Dioscoreae Oppositae (*Shan Yao*), 20g
Semen Coicis Lachryma-jobi (*Yi Yi Ren*), 5g
Fructus Schizandrae Chinensis (*Wu Wei Zi*), 5g
Semen Cuscutae (*Tu Si Zi*), 20g
Semen Allii Tuberosi (*Jiu Zi*), 10g
Fructus Psoraleae Corylifoliae (*Bu Gu Zhi*), 5g
Radix Praeparatus Aconiti Carmichaeli (*Zhi Fu Zi*), 3g
Rhizoma Atractylodis Macrocephalae (*Bai Zhu*), 10g
Semen Litchi Chinensis (*Li Zhi He*), 20g
Semen Citri (*Ju He*), 20g
Fructus Meliae Toosendanis (*Chuan Lian Zi*), 10g
Rhizoma Recens Zingiberis (*Sheng Jiang*), 30g

4. *Shi re xia zhu*
Damp heat pouring downward

Pathognomic manifestations: Swelling of the scrotum and testes accompanied by redness, inflammation, and pain, painful urination, a red tongue with yellow coating, and a rapid, sodden pulse

Therapeutic principles: Clear heat and disinhibit dampness, disperse swelling and stop pain

Guiding formula: *Yi Mi Zhu Ye San Jia Wei*

Semen Coicis Lachryma-jobi (*Yi Yi Ren*), 12g
Stigmata Zeae Maydis (*Yu Mi Xu*), 9g
Herba Lophatheri Gracilis (*Zhu Ye*), 12g
Fructus Meliae Toosendanis (*Chuan Lian Zi*), 10g
Pericarpium Viridis Citri Reticulatae (*Qing Pi*), 10g
Pericarpium Citri Reticulatae (*Chen Pi*), 10g
Fructus Foeniculi Vulgaris (*Xiao Hui Xiang*), 9g
Fructus Kochiae Scopariae (*Di Fu Zi*)

Radix Salviae Miltiorrhizae (*Dan Shen*), 10g
Talcum (*Hua Shi*), 15g
Semen Citri (*Ju He*), 15g

5. *Yin xu*
Yin vacuity

Pathognomic manifestations: Swelling of the scrotum and testes on one or both sides, possible urinary dysfunction, heat in the five centers, night sweats, dizziness, tinnitus, low back and knee soreness and weakness, a red tongue with scant coating, and a thready, rapid pulse

Therapeutic principles: Enrich yin and clear heat, seep dampness and disperse swelling

Guiding formula: *Zhu Ling Tang Jia Wei*

Sclerotium Polypori Umbellati (*Zhu Ling*)
Sclerotium Poriae Cocoris (*Fu Ling*)
Rhizoma Alismatis (*Ze Xie*)
Gelatinum Corii Asini (*E Jiao*)
Talcum (*Hua Shi*)
Semen Citri (*Ju He*)
Semen Litchi Chinensis (*Li Zhi He*)
Fructus Meliae Toosendanis (*Chuan Lian Zi*)

Yun gao zheng
Cryptorchidism

If one or both testicles remain within the inguinal canal inside the abdomen and fail to descend into the scrotum this is called cryptorchidism in modern Western medicine, or hidden testes. If left untreated, this condition may lead to sterility. Since this condition is usually unilateral, it is traditionally called *du shen* or solitary kidney in Chinese, remembering that the testes are often called the *wai shen* or external kidneys. Cryptorchidism is most commonly seen amongst children.

Bing yin bing ji
Disease causes, disease mechanisms

TCM theory posits that this condition is primarily due to kidney qi insufficiency based on the fact that the testes are seen as an external extension or manifestation of the kidneys.

Bian zheng lun zhi
Treatment based on pattern discrimination

1. *Shen qi bu zu*
Kidney qi insufficiency

Pathognomic manifestations: Nondescension of the testicles, poor development of the scrotal area, malnutrition, a thin, white tongue coating, and a thready pulse

Therapeutic principles: Supplement the kidneys and boost the *jing*

Guiding formula:

Radix Coquitus Rehmanniae (*Shu Di Huang*), 6g
Herba Cistanchis (*Rou Cong Rong*), 6g
Herba Epimedii (*Xian Ling Pi*), 6g
Radix Morindae Officinalis (*Ba Ji Tian*), 6g
Semen Astragali (*Sha Yuan Ji Li*), 6g
Semen Cuscutae (*Tu Si Zi*), 12g
Concha Ostreae (*Sheng Mu Li*), 15g
Cortex Cinnamomi (*Rou Gui*), 1.5g
Semen Cnidii Monnieri (*She Chuang Zi*), 4.5g

This condition may require as many as 50 *ji* (literally "prescriptions" but practically meaning "packets").

Jing suo bing
Variocele

Obstruction of the venous return within the scrotum results in variocele. In this case, the local veins will be enlarged, twisted, and will protrude. If the condition is mild, the patient may have no subjective complaints. Occasionally, if this condition becomes bothersome, the patient will complain of a heavy sensation in their scrotum and pain in their scrotum and lower abdomen. These symptoms are typically aggravated by standing or walking for a long time, and bed rest may help alleviate the problem.

Bing yin bing ji
Disease causes, disease mechanisms

According to TCM theory, variocele is mostly the result of liver/kidney vacuity, cold damp obstruction, and qi stagnation and blood stasis. Vacuity of the liver and kidneys may lead to easy accumulation of cold and dampness in the inguinal and scrotal regions. This then obstructs the free and patent flow of qi and blood leading to qi stagnation and blood stasis. This condition can also be complicated by qi vacuity, yang vacuity, yin vacuity with vacuity fire, and damp heat similar to various other of the scrotal diseases described above.

Bian zheng lun zhi
Treatment based on pattern discrimination

A single formula may be used to treat variocele associated with various complicating patterns. This base or guiding formula is designed to nourish liver blood and supplement kidney yang while also activating the blood and transforming stasis.

Guiding formula: Li Jing Jian

Radix Salviae Miltiorrhizae (Dan Shen)

Rhizoma Curcumae Zedoariae (*E Zhu*)
Radix Cyathulae (*Chuan Niu Xi*)
Polyphagae Seu Opisthoplatiae (*Tu Bie Chong*)
Apex Radicis Angelicae Sinensis (*Dang Gui Wei*)
Radix Coquitus Rehmanniae (*Shu Di Huang*)
Radix Dipsaci (*Chuan Xu Duan*)
Fructus Lycii Chinensis (*Gou Qi*)
Herba Epimedii (*Xian Ling Pi*)
Herba Cistanchis (*Rou Cong Rong*)
Cornu Degelatinum Cervi (*Lu Jiao Shuang*)
Fructus Zizyphi Jujubae (*Hong Zao*)

Additions:

For liver channel qi stagnation with a wiry pulse, add:

Semen Citri (*Ju He*)
Folium Citri Reticulatae (*Ju Ye*)
Semen Litchi Chinensis (*Li Zhi He*)
Fructus Foeniculi Vulgaris (*Xiao Hui Xiang*)

For qi vacuity with a thready, weak pulse, add:

Radix Astragali Seu Hedysari (*Huang Qi*)
Radix Codonopsis Pilosulae (*Dang Shen*)
Rhizoma Atractylodis Macrocephalae (*Bai Zhu*)

For yang vacuity with cold limbs and a deep, slow pulse, add:

Radix Praeparatus Aconiti Carmichaeli (*Fu Zi*)
Ramulus Cinnamomi (*Gui Zhi*)

For yin vacuity with stirring of vacuity fire and a thready, rapid pulse, add:

Radix Rehmanniae (*Sheng Di*)
Radix Linderae Strychnifoliae (*Ta Wu Yao*)

Carapax Praeparatus Amydae (*Zhi Bie Jia*)

For damp heat with a yellow, slimy tongue coating and a rapid, sodden pulse, add:

Cortex Phellodendri (*Huang Bai*)
Semen Plantaginis (*Che Qian Zi*)

邪之所凑，其氣必虛。

『素問·評熱病論』

If evil invades, one's qi will become vacuous.

5

Za Bing Miscellaneous Diseases

Qian lie xian yan
Prostatitis

Prostatitis is a modern Western disease category. It refers to either acute or chronic inflammation of the prostate gland. During the acute stage, the commonly encountered signs and symptoms include frequent, urgent, painful urination, genital pain radiating to the inguinal and lower abdominal regions, fever, aversion to cold, and headache and body aches and pains. During the chronic stage, there may be difficulty, frequency, urgency, or painful urination. Additionally, there may be a white discharge at the end of urination, genital pain radiating to the groin or lower abdomen, hypertrophy of the prostate gland, and other such complications. Typically, acute prostatitis is equivalent to *re lin* or hot *lin*.[1] Chronic prostatitis, on the other hand, corresponds to either *lao lin,* taxation *lin*, or *qi lin*.

Bing yin bing ji
Disease causes, disease mechanisms

According to TCM theory, acute prostatitis is due to damp heat pouring down into the lower burner. We have discussed the causes of such damp heat above, under other disease categories. In terms

---

[1] *Lin* diseases are a traditional Chinese disease category characterized by urinary strangury, pain, and/or dribbling. Within the traditional literature, there are a number of types of *lin*.

of chronic prostatitis, this is most often due to cold damp obstruction associated with the liver/kidney vacuity attendant upon aging. In both acute and chronic prostatitis, qi stagnation and blood stasis due to long term obstruction typically play a part, since even acute prostatitis is mostly encountered in middle-aged and older men.

Bian zheng lun zhi
Treatment based on pattern discrimination

1. Shi re xia zhu
Damp heat pouring downward

Pathognomic manifestations: Urinary pain, frequency, urgency, pain in the genitalia radiating to the groin and lower abdomen, fever, headache, body aches and pain, aversion to cold, a red tongue with yellow, slimy coating or a thick yellowish white coating, and a rapid, slippery or sodden pulse

Therapeutic principles: Clear heat and disinhibit dampness, activate the blood and transform stasis

Guiding formula:

Semen Vaccariae Segetalis (*Wang Bu Liu Xing*) 25g
Cortex Phellodendri (*Huang Bai*), 25g
Herba Patriniae Heterophyllae (*Bai Jiang Cao*), 25g
Herba Cum Radice Taraxaci Mongolici (*Pu Gong Ying*), 25g
Radix Rubrus Paeoniae Lactiflorae (*Chi Shao*), 15g
Rhizoma Corydalis Yanhusuo (*Yan Hu*), 15g
Cortex Radicis Moutan (*Dan Pi*), 15g
Squama Manitis (*Chuan Shan Jia*), 15g
Spina Gleditschiae Chinensis (*Chao Jiao Ci*), 15g
Radix Saussureae Seu Vladimiriae (*Mu Xiang*), 10g
Radix Glycyrrhizae (*Gan Cao*), 5-10g

2. *Shen qi xu jia shi zuo*
Kidney qi vacuity plus damp turbidity

Pathognomic manifestations: Chronic urinary frequency, urgency, and pain, a whitish discharge at the end of urination, terminal dribbling, possible pain in the genitals radiating to the groin and/or lower abdomen, a pale, fat tongue with thickish white, slimy coating, and a deep, sodden, wiry pulse

Therapeutic principles: Consolidate the *jing* and lead out turbidity

Guiding formula:

Rhizoma Dioscoreae Hypoglaucae (*Bi Xie*)
Semen Cuscutae (*Tu Si Zi*)
Radix Achyranthis Bidentatae (*Niu Xi*)
Sclerotium Poriae Cocoris (*Fu Ling*)
Rhizoma Alismatis (*Ze Xie*)
Semen Plantaginis (*Che Qian Zi*)
Radix Linderae Strychnifoliae (*Tai Wu Yao*)
Rhizoma Acori Graminei (*Shi Chang Pu*)
Herba Verbenae (*Ma Pian Cao*)
Radix Glycyrrhizae (*Gan Cao*)
Semen Astragali (*Sha Yuan Zi*)
Fructus Alpiniae Oxyphyllae (*Yi Zhi Ren*)
Radix Dioscoreae Oppositae (*Shan Yao*)

Acupuncture/moxibustion therapy

Acupuncture treatment

Needle *Hui Yin* (CV 1) and *Shen Shu* (Bl 23), without retaining the needle, 1 time per day or 1 time every other day. 10 treatments constitute 1 course of treatment.

Acupuncture and moxibustion

Needle *Zhong Ji* (CV 3), *Guan Yuan* (CV 4), *Tai Xi* (Ki 3), *Tai Chong* (Liv 3), and *Hui Yin* (CV 1). Use even technique and retain the needles after the qi has been obtained. Then moxa *Zhong Ji* and *Guan Yuan* directly, 3 cones apiece, or indirectly moxa *Hui Yin* with a moxa pole for 15-30 minutes. Treat once every other day.

Ear acupuncture

Prostate Gland, Bladder, External Genitals, and Adrenals

Qian lie xian fei da
Benign prostatic hypertrophy

Benign prostatic hypertrophy typically results in reduced and astringent urinary stream with increased frequency and terminal dribbling in middle-aged to elderly men. The onset of this condition is usually gradual with symptoms continually increasing in severity. Other symptoms include nocturia and urinary obstruction. All of these symptoms may be aggravated by exposure to cold, waiting too long before voiding the urine, and alcohol consumption. In the early stage, this condition is equivalent to the traditional Chinese disease category *ye niao zheng duo zheng*, increasing frequency of nocturia. In the midstage, this condition corresponds to *niao bi* or urinary obstruction. In the late stage where there is marked urgency and polyuria, this corresponds to *lin zheng* or *lin* pathocondition.

Bing yin bing ji
Disease causes, disease mechanisms

Modern practitioners of TCM regard most cases of benign prostatic hypertrophy to be due in part to blood stasis. This corresponds directly to the physical hypertrophy as described by modern Western medicine. However, depending upon an individual patient's signs and symptoms, their disease mechanisms can also include qi vacuity, yang vacuity, and qi stagnation. Qi vacuity may involve the kidneys alone or the spleen and kidneys. In either case, such vacuity and insufficiency fails to promote the transportation and transformation of body fluids which then accumulate in the bladder. Such vacuity is primarily due to age, but may also be associated with chronic illness, and may be aggravated by faulty diet, such as overeating cold raw foods and drinking cold liquids with meals. Further, emotional frustration may cause liver qi stagnation. Because the liver controls coursing and discharge, and because the liver traverses the genitalia, such qi stagnation may restrict the free and patent flow of qi and thus also water.

Bian zheng lun zhi
Treatment based on pattern discrimination

1. *Xue yu*
Blood stasis

Pathognomic manifestations: Decreased urinary flow or urinary obstruction, nocturia, pain in the perineal area especially after sitting for a long time, a purplish tongue or purple spots or patches on the tongue, a deep and/or grating/astringent pulse

Therapeutic principles: Activate the blood and transform stasis, soften the hard and disinhibit dampness

Guiding formula: *Tao Hong Si Wu Tang Jia Wei* a.k.a. *Hu Po Si Wu Tang*

Radix Coquitus Rehmanniae (*Shu Di*)
Radix Albus Paeoniae Lactiflorae (*Bai Shao*)
Rhizoma Ligustici Wallichii (*Chuan Xiong*)
Radix Angelicae Sinensis (*Dang Gui*)
Semen Pruni Persicae (*Tao Ren*)

Flos Carthami Tinctorii (*Hong Hua*)
Radix Achyranthis Bidentatae (*Niu Xi*)
Radix Salviae Miltiorrhizae (*Dan Shen*)
Squama Manitis (*Chuan Shan Jia*)
Cortex Cinnamomi (*Rou Gui*)
Succinum (*Hu Po*)
Semen Vaccariae Segetalis (*Wang Bu Liu Xing*)

Additions:

If yang vacuity complicates this condition, add:

Radix Praeparatus Aconiti Carmichaeli (*Fu Zi*)

If qi stagnation complicates this condition, add:

Radix Linderae Strychnifoliae (*Tai Wu Yao*)
Fructus Foeniculi Vulgaris (*Xiao Hui Xiang*)

If there is urinary blockage or obstruction, add:

Medulla Tetrapanacis Papyriferi (*Tong Cao*)
Rhizoma Alismatis (*Ze Xie*)
Radix Platycodi Grandiflori (*Jie Geng*)

2. *Pi shen liang xu*
   Spleen/kidney dual vacuity

Pathognomic manifestations: Urinary frequency, urgency, incontinence, and terminal dribbling, cold extremities and especially the feet, fatigue, low back soreness and weakness, possible digestive complaints, loose stools and/or constipation, a pale, possibly fat tongue with a thin, white coating, and a thready, weak pulse

Therapeutic principles: Supplement the kidneys and strengthen the spleen

Guiding formula:

Radix Praeparatus Astragali Seu Hedysari (*Zhi Huang Qi*), 15g
Radix Codonopsis Pilosulae (*Dang Shen*), 15g
Radix Dioscoreae Oppositae (*Shan Yao*), 15g
Radix Dipsaci (*Chuan Xu Duan*), 15g
Ramus Loranthi Seu Visci (*Sang Ji Sheng*), 15g
Sclerotium Poriae Cocoris (*Fu Ling*), 15g
Rhizoma Alismatis (*Ze Xie*), 10g
Cortex Radicis Moutan (*Dan Pi*), 10g
Radix Linderae Strychnifoliae (*Tai Wu Yao*), 15g
Fructus Rubi (*Fu Pen Zi*), 15g

3. *Gan yu qi zhi*
Liver depression, qi stagnation:

Pathognomic manifestations: Urinary strangury and obstruction which becomes worse when stressed or frustrated, lower abdominal distention, possible flatulence, a normal or slightly dark tongue with inflated rims, and a wiry pulse

Therapeutic principles: Course the liver and regulate the qi, soften the hard and seep dampness

Guiding formula: *Shu Gan San Jie Fang*

Radix Bupleuri (*Chai Hu*)
Radix Salviae Miltiorrhizae (*Dan Shen*)
Radix Rubrus Paeoniae Lactiflorae (*Chi Shao*)
Radix Angelicae Sinensis (*Dang Gui*)
Radix Achyranthis Bidentatae (*Niu Xi*)
Concha Ostreae (*Sheng Mu Li*)
Radix Scrophulariae Ningpoensis (*Yuan Shen*)
Bulbus Fritillariae Cirrhosae (*Chuan Bei Mu*)
Spica Prunellae Vulgaris (*Xia Gu Cao*)
Herba Sargassi (*Hai Zao*)
Thallus Algae (*Kun Bu*)
Pumice (*Hai Fu Shi*)

Nan zi bu yu
Male infertility

Male infertility in Chinese medicine is defined as inability to foster conception after having intercourse without using birth control with the same sex partner for two years or more. According to modern Western medicine some of the causes of male infertility include impotence, premature ejaculation, spermatorrhea, failure to ejaculate, scrotal inflammation, prostatitis, sperm malformation or malfunction, maldevelopment of the sex organs, poor nutrition, injury, and emotional problems. A number of these pathoconditions have been discussed above under various chapters and headings.

Bing yin bing ji
Disease causes, disease mechanisms

Since the semen is called the *sheng zhi zhi jing* or reproductive essence and the *jing* is stored in the kidneys, and since it is also said that kidney *jing* governs birth, growth, maturation, and decline, TCM tends to emphasize the role of the kidneys and *jing* essence in both male and female infertility. Although *jing* is spoken of as yin in comparison to qi which is yang, *jing* can, in fact, be seen as yin or yang depending upon the circumstance. Therefore, kidney yin or yang vacuity can result in *jing* insufficiency. Kidney vacuity is typically due to aging, chronic disease, taxation, drug use, and congenital insufficiency.

However, there are two types of *jing* essence. Although the reproductive essence is associated with the kidney *jing* or *xian tian zhi jing*, this is nourished and bolstered by the acquired or *hou tian zhi jing*. The spleen and stomach are the root of qi and blood production. Each day they manufacture qi and blood from the refined essence of food and drink. If one manufactures more qi and blood than they consume in a day, at night, during deep sleep, this excess qi and blood is transformed into acquired *jing* to also be stored in the kidneys. Therefore, qi and blood vacuity due to either poor diet, taxation, or spleen and stomach dysfunction can also lead to infertility due to a lack of acquired *jing* nourishing and supporting the congenital *jing*.

Even if the *jing* essence is sufficient or nearly so, it may still be blocked and obstructed. The types of evil qi which may hinder the free flow of *jing* are qi stagnation due to liver depression, blood stasis, phlegm dampness, and damp heat. Liver qi stagnation is primarily due to emotional stress and frustration. Blood stasis may be due to long term qi stagnation or past trauma. Phlegm dampness is mostly due to congenital constitution plus faulty diet, and damp heat may be due to faulty diet alone or a combination of faulty diet and emotional stress transforming into evil heat.

Bian zheng lun zhi
Treatment based on pattern discrimination

1. *Shen jing bu zu*
Kidney essence insufficiency

Pathognomic manifestations: Infertility, general debility, tendency to catch cold, vision and hearing problems, forgetfulness or lack of mental clarity, fatigue, low back and knee soreness and weakness, a pale, flaccid tongue, and deep, weak, thready pulse

Therapeutic principles: Supplement the kidneys and boost the *jing*

Guiding formulas:

Wu Zi Heng Zhong Wan

Fructus Lycii Chinensis (*Gou Qi Zi*)
Semen Cuscutae (*Tu Si Zi*)
Fructus Schizandrae Chinensis (*Wu Wei Zi*)
Fructus Rubi (*Fu Pen Zi*)
Semen Plantaginis (*Che Qian Zi*)

Qi Bao Mei Su Dan

Radix Polygoni Multiflori (*He Shou Wu*), 300g
Sclerotium Poriae Cocoris (*Fu Ling*), 150g
Radix Achyranthis Bidentatae (*Niu Xi*), 150g
Radix Angelicae Sinensis (*Dang Gui*), 150g
Fructus Lycii Chinensis (*Gou Qi Zi*), 150g
Semen Cuscutae (*Tu Si Zi*), 150g
Fructus Psoraleae Corylifoliae (*Bu Gu Zhi*), 120g

Grind the above ingredients into powder and make into pills with honey. The normal dose is 1 pill in the morning and evening with warm water.

2. Shen yang xu
Kidney yang vacuity

Pathognomic manifestations: Infertility, diminished sex drive, spermatorrhea, polyuria, nocturia, low back and knee soreness and weakness, dizziness and tinnitus, cold lower extremities, a pale tongue with thin, white coating, and a deep, slow pulse

Therapeutic principles: Supplement the kidneys, warm yang, and boost the *jing*

Guiding formulas:

You Gui Wan (see above)

Zan Yu Dan

Radix Coquitus Rehmanniae (*Shu Di*)
Rhizoma Atractylodis Macrocephalae (*Bai Zhu*)
Radix Angelicae Sinensis (*Dang Gui*)
Fructus Lycii Chinensis (*Gou Qi Zi*)
Cortex Eucommiae Ulmoidis (*Du Zhong*)
Rhizoma Curculiginis Orchoidis (*Xian Mao*)

Fructus Corni Officinalis (*Shan Yu Rou*)
Herba Epimedii (*Yin Yang Huo*)
Herba Cistanchis (*Rou Cong Rong*)
Semen Allii Tuberosi (*Jiu Cai Zi*)
Semen Cnidii Monnieri (*She Chuan Zi*)
Radix Praeparatus Aconiti Carmichaeli (*Fu Zi*)
Cortex Cinnamomi (*Rou Gui*)

Da Tu Si Zi Wan

Semen Cuscutae (*Tu Si Zi*)
Fructus Ligustri Lucidi (*Nu Zhen Zi*)
Fructus Lycii Chinensis (*Gou Qi Zi*)
Radix Polygoni Multiflori (*He Shou Wu*)
Radix Coquitus Rehmanniae (*Shu Di Huang*)
Fructus Corni Officinalis (*Shan Yu Rou*)
Herba Ecliptae Prostratae (*Han Lian Cao*)
Fructus Mori Albi (*Sang Shen*)
Fructus Psoraleae Corylifoliae (*Bu Gu Zhi*)
Herba Cistanchis (*Rou Cong Rong*)

3. Shen yin xu
Kidney yin vacuity

Pathognomic manifestations: Infertility, spermatorrhea, premature ejaculation, polyuria, nocturia, dizziness, tinnitus, low back and knee soreness and weakness, heat in the five centers, heart palpitations, night sweats, a red tongue with scant coating, and a deep, thready, rapid pulse

Therapeutic principles: Supplement the kidneys, enrich yin, and fulfill the *jing*

Guiding formulas:

Liu Wei Di Huang Wan (see above)

Da Bu Yin Wan (see above)

Zuo Gui Wan

Radix Coquitus Rehmanniae (*Shu Di*)
Radix Dioscoreae Oppositae (*Shan Yao*)
Fructus Lycii Chinensis (*Gou Qi*)
Fructus Corni Officinalis (*Shan Zhu Yu*)
Semen Cuscutae (*Tu Si Zi*)
Radix Cyathulae (*Chuan Niu Xi*)
Colla Cornu Cervi (*Lu Jiao Jiao*)
Colla Plastri Testudinis (*Gui Ban Jiao*)

Zhi Bai Di Huang Wan (see above)

4. *Xue yu jing xu*
   Blood stasis, *jing* vacuity

Pathognomic manifestations: Infertility with a long history of qi stagnation or a past history of trauma to the genitals or lower abdomen, withered or dusky complexion, dry skin, varicose veins, low back soreness and weakness, lower abdominal pain, a pale tongue with possible ecchymotic spots or patches, and a deep, thready, wiry pulse

Therapeutic principles: Activate the blood and nourish the *jing*

Guiding formulas:

Tao Hong Si Wu Tang (see above)

Xue Fu Zhu Yu Tang (see above)

Shi Xiao San

Feces Trogopterori Seu Pteromi (*Wu Ling Zhi*)
Pollen Typhae (*Pu Huang*)

This last formula may be added to other formulas if there is blood stasis accompanied by pain. If there are pronounced signs and symptoms of kidney vacuity plus blood stasis, then use:

Shen Qi Wan (see above) plus:

Squama Manitis (*Chuan Shan Jia*)
Semen Vaccariae Segetalis (*Wang Bu Liu Xing*)
Fructus Liquidambaris Taiwanianae (*Lu Lu Tong*)
Radix Achyranthis Bidentatae (*Niu Xi*)

If the *jing* palace is blocked by dampness and stasis, then use:

Rhizoma Dioscoreae Hypoglaucae (*Bi Xie*)
Sclerotium Poriae Cocoris (*Fu Ling*)
Semen Coicis Lachryma-jobi (*Yi Yi Ren*)
Semen Plantaginis (*Che Qian Zi*)
Rhizoma Alismatis (*Ze Xie*)
Semen Pruni Persicae (*Tao Ren*)
Herba Leonuri Heterophylli (*Yi Mu Cao*)
Radix Rubrus Paeoniae Lactiflorae (*Chi Shao*)
Flos Carthami Tinctorii (*Hong Hua*)
Rhizoma Acori Graminei (*Shi Chang Pu*)

5. Gan qi yu jing bu zu
Liver qi depression, jing insufficiency

Pathognomic manifestations: Infertility, emotional depression, irritability, chest oppression, flank pain, low back and knee soreness and weakness, dizziness, tinnitus, poor memory, dry skin, lack of lustre in the facial complexion, a pale, somewhat dark tongue with swollen rims and thin, white coating, and a thready, wiry pulse

Therapeutic principles: Course the liver and regulate the qi, resolve depression and nourish the kidneys

Guiding formulas:

Unnamed formula

Radix Bupleuri (*Chai Hu*)
Radix Linderae Strychnifoliae (*Tai Wu Yao*)
Semen Citri (*Ju He*)
Lignum Aquilariae Agallochae (*Chen Xiang*)
Radix Albus Paeoniae Lactiflorae (*Bai Shao*)
Radix Angelicae Sinensis (*Dang Gui*)
Herba Epimedii (*Yin Yang Huo*)
Rhizoma Curculiginis Orchoidis (*Xian Mao*)
Rhizoma Cyperi Rotundi (*Xiang Fu*)
Radix Glycyrrhizae (*Gan Cao*)

Xiao Yao San (see above)

Si Ni San (see above)

Chai Hu Shu Gan San (see above)

If cold stasis is obstructing the liver channel, then use:

Nuan Gan Jian (see above)

Dang Gui Si Ni Tang (see above)

Tian Tai Wu Yao San

Radix Linderae Strychnifoliae (*Tai Wu Yao*)
Radix Saussureae Seu Vladimiriae (*Mu Xiang*)
Fructus Foeniculi Vulgaris (*Xiao Hui Xiang*)
Pericarpium Viridis Citri Reticulatae (*Qing Pi*)
Rhizoma Alpiniae Officinari (*Gao Liang Jiang*)
Semen Arecae Catechu (*Bing Lang*)
Fructus Meliae Toosendanis (*Chuan Lian Zi*)
Semen Crotonis Tiglii (*Ba Dou*)

6. *Tan shi zu yao jing shi*
Phlegm dampness obstructing the palace of *jing*

Pathognomic manifestations: Infertility coupled with obesity, excessive phlegm production, stuffy chest and epigastrium, heaviness of the body and head, damp scrotum, possible loose stools, an enlarged tongue with teeth indentations and a white, slimy coating, and a sodden or slippery, wiry pulse

Therapeutic principles: Transform phlegm and eliminate dampness to clear the essence palace

Guiding formulas:

Ping Wei San

Rhizoma Atractylodis (*Cang Zhu*)
Cortex Magnoliae Officinalis (*Hou Po*)
Pericarpium Citri Reticulatae (*Chen Pi*)
Radix Glycyrrhizae (*Gan Cao*)
Rhizoma Recens Zingiberis (*Sheng Jiang*)
Fructus Zizyphi Jujubae (*Da Zao*)

plus *Er Chen Tang* (see above)

plus *Cang Fu Dao Tan Wan*

Rhizoma Atractylodis (*Cang Zhu*)
Radix Praeparatus Aconiti Carmichaeli (*Fu Zi*)
Rhizoma Pinelliae Ternatae (*Ban Xia*)
Pericarpium Citri Erythrocarpae (*Ju Hong*)
Sclerotium Poriae Cocoris (*Fu Ling*)
Rhizoma Praeparata Cum Fellem Bovim Arisaematis (*Dan Nan Xing*)
Fructus Immaturus Citri Seu Ponciri (*Zhi Shi*)
Radix Praeparatus Glycyrrhizae (*Zhi Gan Cao*)

7. *Shi re xia zhu*
Damp heat pouring downward

Pathognomic manifestations: Infertility, spermatorrhea, premature ejaculation, occasional dysuria, occasional or possible genital sores, possible bloody semen, itching and wet rash in the groin or on the lower extremities, possible constipation or diarrhea, a red tongue with a yellow coating, and a rapid, sodden pulse

Therapeutic principles: Clear heat and disinhibit dampness

Guiding formulas:

Long Dan Xie Gan Tang (see above)

San Miao San (see above)

San Ren Tang (see above)

8. *Qi xue xu*
Qi & blood vacuity

Pathognomic manifestations: Infertility, a pale face, fatigue, shortness of breath, dizziness, tinnitus, lack of strength in the extremities, a pale tongue with thin, white coating, and a thready, weak pulse

Therapeutic principles: Supplement the qi, nourish the blood, and fulfill the *jing*

Guiding formulas:

Selection of a guiding formula for this pattern depends upon whether qi vacuity is more pronounced or blood vacuity is more pronounced and also the state of the digestion or middle burner.

If qi vacuity and *jing* insufficiency predominate, use:

Liu Jun Zi Tang

Radix Panacis Ginseng (*Ren Shen*)
Rhizoma Atractylodis Macrocephalae (*Bai Zhu*)
Sclerotium Poriae Cocoris (*Fu Ling*)
Pericarpium Citri Reticulatae (*Chen Pi*)
Rhizoma Pinelliae Ternatae (*Ban Xia*)
Radix Praeparatus Glycyrrhizae (*Zhi Gan Cao*)

plus **Wu Zi Heng Zhong Wan** (see above)

For pronounced qi vacuity of the middle burner, use:

Bu Zhong Yi Qi Tang (see above).

For spleen vacuity which has become yang vacuity, use:

Li Zhong Wan

Radix Panacis Ginseng (*Ren Shen*)
Rhizoma Atractylodis Macrocephalae (*Bai Zhu*)
Rhizoma Desiccata Zingiberis (*Gan Jiang*)
Radix Praeparatus Glycyrrhizae (*Zhi Gan Cao*)

If one adds Radix Praeparatus Aconiti Carmichaeli and Cortex Cinnamomi (*Rou Gui*), this becomes **Fu Zi Li Zhong Wan.**

If blood and *jing* are both vacuous and insufficient, then use:

Gui Pi Tang (see above)

Si Wu Tang

Radix Coquitus Rehmanniae (*Shu Di*)
Radix Albus Paeoniae Lactiflorae (*Bai Shao*)

Radix Angelicae Sinensis (*Dang Gui*)
Rhizoma Ligustici Wallichii (*Chuan Xiong*)

Wu Zi Heng Zhong Wan (see above)

If both qi and blood are vacuous and insufficient, use:

Ba Zhen Tang

Radix Panacis Ginseng (*Ren Shen*)
Rhizoma Atractylodis Macrocephalae (*Bai Zhu*)
Sclerotium Poriae Cocoris (*Fu Ling*)
Radix Praeparatus Glycyrrhizae (*Zhi Gan Cao*)
Radix Angelicae Sinensis (*Dang Gui*)
Radix Coquitus Rehmanniae (*Shu Di*)
Radix Albus Paeoniae Lactiflorae (*Bai Shao*)
Rhizoma Ligustici Wallichii (*Chuan Xiong*)

Shi Quan Da Bu Wan (see above)

Acupuncture/moxibustion therapy

Main points: *Shen Shu* (Bl 23), *Ci Liao* (Bl 32), *Guan Yuan* (CV 4), and *Qi Chong* (ST 30)

Additions:

For impotence, add *Zu San Li* (St 36) and *Tai Xi* (Ki 3).

For failure to ejaculate, add, *San Yin Jiao* (Sp 6), *Tai Chong* (Liv 3), and *Yin Ling Quan* (Sp 9).

For malformation of the sperm, add *Zu San Li* (St 36), *Tai Chong* (Liv 3), *Tai Xi* (Ki 3), *Ming Men* (GV 4), and *Hua Tuo Jia Ji* points along the lumbar spine

Shu hou zong he zheng
Complications of vasectomy

Recent Western research suggests that there is an increased incidence of prostate cancer in men who have undergone vasectomies. TCM theory and practice supports this idea. Based on clinical experience in China, vasectomies tend to create or aggravate qi stagnation and blood stasis. This then can cause or complicate such conditions as scrotal inflammation, severe pain of the scrotum, groin, and lower abdomen, and testicular swelling and pain. Typically, these complications arise directly after surgery. However, they suggest that vasectomies may indeed have long term negative effects on the genitourinary organs.

For improved healing post-surgery, one can use **Tao He Cheng Qi Tang Jia Wei** in order to prevent the above complicating sequelae.

Semen Pruni Persicae (*Tao Ren*)
Ramulus Cinnamomi (*Gui Zhi*)
Radix Et Rhizoma Rhei (*Da Huang*)
Mirabilitum (*Mang Xiao*)
Radix Praeparatus Glycyrrhizae (*Zhi Gan Cao*)
Semen Litchi Chinensis (*Li Zhi He*)
Fructus Crataegi (*Shan Zha*)
Flos Carthami Tinctorii (*Hong Hua*)
Fructus Foeniculi Vulgaris (*Xiao Hui Xiang*)

One can also use:

Long Dan Er He Tao Hong Gan Cao Tang.

Radix Gentianae Scabrae (*Long Dan Cao*), 20g
Semen Litchi Chinensis (*Li Zhi He*), 10g
Semen Citri (*Ju He*), 10g
Semen Pruni Persicae (*Tao Ren*), 10g
Flos Carthami Tinctorii (*Hong Hua*), 3g

Radix Glycyrrhizae (*Gan Cao*), 3g

Additions:

For scrotal inflammation, add:

Fructus Gardeniae Jasminoidis (*Zhi Zi*)
Radix Scutellariae Baicalensis (*Huang Qin*)
Cortex Phellodendri (*Huang Bai*)
Flos Lonicerae Japonicae (*Yin Hua*)

For severe pain, add:

Rhizoma Sparganii (*San Leng*)
Rhizoma Curcumae Zedoariae (*E Zhu*)
Rhizoma Ligustici Wallichii (*Chuan Xiong*)
Fructus Foeniculi Vulgaris (*Xiao Hui Xiang*)
Concha Ostreae (*Mu Li*)

For testicular swelling and pain, add:

Herba Agrimoniae Pilosae (*Xian He Cao*)
Radix Rubiae Cordifoliae (*Qian Ca Geng*)
Radix Pseudoginseng (*San Qi*)
Gelatinum Corii Asini (*E Jiao*)
Radix Rehmanniae (*Sheng Di*)
Cortex Radicis Moutan (*Dan Pi*)

Acupuncture/moxibustion therapy

Main points: *Ah Si* points plus *Qi Hai* (CV 6) and *Xia Wan* (CV 10)

Additions:

For qi stagnation, add: *Shan Zhong* (CV 17)

For blood stasis, add: *Ge Shu* (Bl 17)

For qi vacuity, add: *Zu San Li* (St 36)

For yang vacuity, add: *Guan Yuan* (CV 4) and *Shen Shu* (Bl 23)

Moxibustion is also applicable.

Nan xing geng nian qu zong he zheng
Male climacteric

The climacteric occurs somewhere between the ages of 55-65 in the adult male. It is that period of time when the middle-aged man is becoming an old man. Although there is no single physiological change or event similar to menopause in females, still, this change in a man's life is fraught with a number of possible imbalances, and this is a time when an otherwise or hitherto healthy male may begin experiencing various diseases.

Bing yin bing ji
Disease causes, disease mechanisms

As stated above, the male climacteric is not a disease *per se* nor is it a syndrome in the way that menopausal syndrome is in women. Nonetheless, one can delineate the main mechanisms responsible for common complaints which may crop up at this time. First of all, the spleen/stomach which has been declining subtly since the late 30s and early 40s may become even more obviously deficient. This may lead to vacuities of either or both the qi and blood. Qi vacuity may then affect any organ in the body but most particularly tends to affect the lungs, spleen, and kidneys. If qi vacuity becomes more pronounced, it may develop into spleen yang or kidney yang vacuity.

Because the blood and *jing* share a common source, blood vacuity may result in liver blood vacuity and/or kidney yin vacuity. This may give rise to flaring of vacuity fire which may disturb the spirit within the heart. The heart spirit may also become disturbed if spleen qi vacuity and heart blood vacuity combine to leave the spirit malnourished within the heart. Since old people often cannot do or do not have to do the work they previously did, a combination of worry and declining digestion aggravate this tendency to heart/spleen dual vacuity with attendant disturbance of the spirit.

If spleen and lung qi declines in function, this may give rise to the generation and accumulation of phlegm and dampness. At the same time, the lungs may also become yin deficient along with the kidneys. This phlegm and dampness and vacuity of the lungs, spleen, and kidneys may cause chronic upper respiratory problems.

In addition, many individuals experience a sense of melancholy and frustration at aging. They cannot do what they have been used to doing and they see only further decline and debility before them. This can be very depressing, and this depression can cause or aggravate liver qi stagnation. This liver qi stagnation may further weaken the spleen, and it may also give rise to blood stasis in various parts of the body, including the chest. Within the chest, such stagnant qi and blood may give rise to pain and eventually heart disease.

Bian zheng lun zhi
Treatment based on pattern discrimination

1. Zhong jiao kui xu
Middle burner deficiency & vacuity

Pathognomic manifestations: Fatigue, palpitations, forgetfulness, spontaneous perspiration, a heavy feeling in the body, shortness of breath, a pale tongue with a thin coating, and a weak pulse

Therapeutic principles: Supplement the middle and boost the qi

Guiding formula: *Huang Qi Jian Zhong Tang* (see above)

2. *Xin qi shen yang xu*
   Heart qi/kidney yang vacuity

Pathognomic manifestations: Palpitations, deafness, blurred vision, itching of the entire body, lower abdominal distention and pain, a pale tongue, and a thready, deep pulse

Therapeutic principles: Supplement the heart and kidneys and assist yang

Guiding formula: *Wai Tai Bu Shen Fang*

Magnetitum (*Ci Shi*), 15g
Rhizoma Recens Zingiberis (*Sheng Jiang*), 10g
Radix Ledebouriellae Sesloidis (*Fang Feng*), 10g
Fructus Schizandrae Chinensis (*Wu Wei Zi*), 10g
Radix Scrophulariae Ningpoensis (*Yuan Shen*), 10g
Cortex Cinnamomi (*Gui Xin*), 10g
Cortex Radicis Moutan (*Dan Pi*), 10g
Semen Germinatus Glycinis (*Da Dou*), 15g
Radix Praeparatus Aconiti Carmichaeli (*Pao Fu Zi*), 6g

3. *Xin shen bu ning*
   Heart spirit not tranquil

Pathognomic manifestations: Depression, restlessness, easily angered, paranoia, dream-disturbed sleep, palpitations, a thin, white tongue coating, and a wiry, thready pulse

Therapeutic principles: Nourish the heart and calm the spirit

Guiding formula: *Gan Mai Da Zao Tang*

Radix Glycyrrhizae (*Gan Cao*), 10g
Fructus Tritici Levis (*Fu Xiao Mai*), 30g

Fructus Zizyphi Jujubae (*Da Zao*), 9g

4. *Fei shen yin xu he tan shi*
Lung/kidney yin vacuity with phlegm dampness

Pathognomic manifestations: Productive cough with white mucous which is difficult to expectorate and may taste salty, nausea, dizziness, blurred vision, bloody stools, a stuffy sensation in the chest, a red tongue with slimy, white coating, and a thready, rapid pulse

Therapeutic principles: Enriches and nourishes the lungs and kidneys, eliminates dampness and transforms phlegm

Guiding formula: *Jin Shui Liu Jun Jian*

Radix Angelicae Sinensis (*Dang Gui*), 10g
Pericarpium Citri Reticulatae (*Chen Pi*), 6g
Rhizoma Pinelliae Ternatae (*Ban Xia*), 10g
Radix Coquitus Rehmanniae (*Shu Di*), 15g
Rhizoma Recens Zingiberis (*Sheng Jiang*), 10g
Radix Praeparatus Glycyrrhizae (*Zhi Gan Cao*), 6g
Sclerotium Poriae Cocoris (*Fu Ling*), 10g

5. *Gan shen liang xu he gan qi zhi*
Liver/kidney dual vacuity with liver qi stagnation

Pathognomic manifestations: Cardiac pain, flank pain, irritability, insomnia, dream-disturbed sleep, dry mouth and parched throat, yellow urine, constipation, a red tongue with scant coating, and a thready, wiry pulse

Therapeutic principles: Harmonize the liver and enrich the kidneys

Guiding formula: *Yi Guan Jian*

Radix Rehmanniae (*Sheng Di*)
Radix Glehniae Littoralis (*Sha Shen*)
Tuber Ophiopogonis Japonicae (*Mai Dong*)
Radix Angelicae Sinensis (*Dang Gui*)
Fructus Lycii Chinensis (*Gou Qi Zi*)
Fructus Meliae Toosendanis (*Chuan Lian Zi*)

6. *Gan yu qi zhi*
Liver depression, qi stagnation

Pathognomic manifestations: Fatigue, lack of appetite, flank distention, dizziness, tinnitus, dry mouth, and a wiry, forceless pulse

Therapeutic principles: Course the liver and regulate the qi, strengthen the spleen and supplement the kidneys

Guiding formula: *Hei Xiao Yao San*

Radix Bupleuri (*Chai Hu*), 9g
Radix Angelicae Sinensis (*Dang Gui*), 12g
Radix Albus Paeoniae Lactiflorae (*Bai Shao*), 10g
Radix Coquitus Rehmanniae (*Shu Di*), 12g
Rhizoma Atractylodis Macrocephalae (*Bai Zhu*), 9g
Sclerotium Poriae Cocoris (*Fu Ling*), 9g
Radix Glycyrrhizae (*Gan Cao*), 3g

Bibliography

Gu Jin Nan Ke Yi An Xuan An (Classic & Modern Case Histories in Urology), Dai Xi-hu & Liu Jian-hua, Hua Xia Press, Beijing, 1990

Nan Ke Zheng Zhi Xin Fa (Heart Methods & Oroven Treatments in Urology), Cheng Shao-en *et al.*, Beijing Science & Technology Press, Beijing, 1991

Nan Nu Bing Mi Yan Liang Fang (Secret, Proven, Fine Formulas for Men's & Women's Disease), Du Jie-hui, Beijing Science & Technology Press, Beijing, 1991

Xian Dai Zhong Yi Nan Ke Hui Cui (A Compilation of Modern Chinese Urology), Wang Yi & Qing Guo-cheng, Hua Xia Press, Beijing, 1990

Xin Gong Nen Zang Ai Yu Zhong Yi Zhe Wo Gan Fu (Sexual Dysfunction & Self-healing with Chinese Medicine), Chao Jia-qi & Xie Xin-ming, Tianjin University Press, Tianjin, 1989

Yi Xin Fang Nan Ke Qi Lan (Curious Readings on Urology from the Heart Formulas of Medicine), Chen He-liang, Hua Xia Press, Beijing, 1991

Zhong Guo Nan Ke Yi An (Chinese Urology Case Histories), Zhang You-yi, Tianjin Science & Technology and Translation Press, Tianjin, 1990

Zhong Yi Lin Chuang Ge Ke (Various Specialties in the Clinical Practice of Chinese Medicine), Zhang En-qin *et. al.*, Shanghai College of TCM Press, Shanghai, 1990

Zhong Yi Nan Ke Bai Wen (One Hundred Questons in Chinese Urology), Wu Yin-geng & Shen Qing-fa, Shanghai Science & Technology Press, Shanghai, 1990

Zhong Yi Nan Ke Lin Chuang Zhi Liao Xue (A Study in the Clinical Treatment of TCM Urology), Leng Fang-nan, People's Health & Hygiene Press, Beijing, 1991

Zhong Yi Nan Ke Ming Fang Xuan Yi (Famous Ancient Chinese Formulas for Urology), Liu Cai-jian, Hua Xia Press, Beijing, 1990

Index

A

abdomen and testicles, cold 100, 147
abdominal spasm 139
addictions 26
aging 13, 19, 23, 24, 51, 86, 95, 101, 108, 137, 172, 186, 192, 206
angered, easily 70, 93, 104, 127, 139, 207
anus 10, 147
appetite, loss of 60, 132
appetite, poor 81
asthma 55, 57, 58
aversion to chill 161
aversion to cold 6, 56, 146, 160, 166, 185, 186
awakened, easily 145
azoospermia 107, 108

B

Ba Wei Di Huang Wan 44-46, 48-50, 97, 98, 148, 156
Ba Zhen Tang 202
Ban Xia Hou Po Tang 47
beng lou 59
benign prostatic hypertrophy 188
Bi Bai Cang Zhu Jian 83
Bi Xie Fen Qing Yin 94, 125, 156
bian zheng lun zhi 17, 53, 68, 77, 86, 89, 96, 101, 108, 110, 114, 116, 119, 138, 140, 142, 144, 145, 147, 153, 156, 157, 158, 159, 161, 166, 170, 172, 175, 180, 181, 186, 189, 193, 206
birth control 192
bitter taste in the mouth 80, 83, 90, 97, 139
blurred vision 129, 138, 207, 208
body aches and pains 185
body odor 68
body, weakness of the entire 132
breath, shortness of 4, 81, 87, 110, 112, 132, 177, 200, 206
bu she jing 88

Bu Shen Yi Qi Tong Jing Tang 93
Bu Zhong Yi Qi Tang 49, 97, 98, 112, 132, 201
Bu Zhong Yi Qi Tang He Wu Zi Yan Zong Tang 112

C

cancer, penile 141
Cang Fu Dao Tan Wan 199
cardiac pain 208
castration 7
cauliflower kidney rocks 141
central nervous system disorders 9
cerebrospinal disease 136
Chai Hu Jia Long Gu Mu Li Tang 46, 48
Chai Hu Shu Gan Tang 126
chest oppression 66, 68, 89, 90, 125, 197
chest pain 90, 93
chest stuffy 133, 134, 156, 199
chilled feet 120
climacteric, male 19, 205
cold hands when nervous 89
cold limbs 6, 56, 100, 182
cold lower extremities 93, 101, 194
cold, tendency to catch 193
coldness, lower abdominal 147
concentrating, difficulty 66
congenital insufficiency 3, 7, 101, 108, 144, 145, 192
constipation 60, 99, 122, 190, 200, 208
cough 6, 57, 58, 133, 173, 208
cough with white mucous 208
cystitis 136

D

Da Bu Yin Wan 79, 92, 138, 196
Da Bu Yuan Jian 131
Da Chai Hu Tang 48
Da Huang Mu Dan Pi Tang 43, 44
Da Tu Si Zi Wan 195
Da Yi Tang 34

About the Author

Anna Lin, MA, Lic. Ac., Dipl. Ac., was born in Cambodia to a Chinese family with a long history of involvement with Chinese medicine. Her first experiences with the art of Chinese medicine came at a very early age. She began by following and learning acupuncture technique from her aunt. Later she apprenticed with a Dr. Ma in Saigon, Vietnam. After that, Ms. Lin studied at the Guangzhou College of Traditional Chinese Medicine in the People's Republic of China and interned at both the Guangzhou TCM Hospital and the Xiamen TCM Hospital. In addition, Ms. Lin received her BA degree in literature and languages from Jinan University in Guangzhou.

During the 1980s, Anna Lin practiced acupuncture and Traditional Chinese Medicine in New Mexico along with earning her MA in American Studies. She currently conducts a private practice in Torrance, CA and is an instructor at both SAMRA University of Oriental Medicine and Yosan University of Oriental Medicine. Ms. Lin also gives CEU seminars to licensed acupuncturists at these two colleges. Besides this book, Anna Lin is the co-author of *The Dao of Increasing Longevity: A Handbook of Traditional Chinese Geriatrics and Chinese Herbal Patent Medicines*.

OTHER BOOKS ON CHINESE MEDICINE AVAILABLE FROM BLUE POPPY PRESS

1775 Linden Ave
Boulder, CO 80304
For ordering 1-800-487-9296
PH. 303\442-0796 FAX 303\447-0740

PMS: Its Cause, Diagnosis & Treatment According to Traditional Chinese Medicine by Bob Flaws ISBN 0-936185-22-8 $14.95

SOMETHING OLD, SOMETHING NEW; Essays on the TCM Description of Western Herbs, Pharmaceuticals, Vitamins & Minerals by Bob Flaws ISBN 0-936185-21-X $19.95

SCATOLOGY & THE GATE OF LIFE: The Role of the Large Intestine in Immunity, An Integrated Chinese-Western Approach by Bob Flaws ISBN 0-936185-20-1 $12.95

SECOND SPRING: A Guide To Healthy Menopause Through Traditional Chinese Medicine by Honora Lee Wolfe ISBN 0-936185-18-X $14.95

MIGRAINES & TRADITIONAL CHINESE MEDICINE: A Layperson's Guide by Bob Flaws ISBN 0-936185-15-5 $11.95

STICKING TO THE POINT: A Rational Methodology for the Step by Step Formulation & Administration of an Acupuncture Treatment by Bob Flaws ISBN 0-936185-17-1 $14.95

ENDOMETRIOSIS & INFERTILITY AND TRADITIONAL CHINESE MEDICINE: A Laywoman's Guide by Bob Flaws ISBN 0-936185-14-7 $9.95

THE BREAST CONNECTION: A Laywoman's Guide to the Treatment of Breast Disease by Chinese Medicine by Honora Lee Wolfe ISBN 0-936185-13-9 $8.95

NINE OUNCES: A Nine Part Program For The Prevention of AIDS in HIV Positive Persons by Bob Flaws ISBN 0-936185-12-0 $9.95

THE TREATMENT OF CANCER BY INTEGRATED CHINESE-WESTERN MEDICINE by Zhang Daizhao, trans. by Zhang Ting-liang & Bob Flaws, ISBN 0-936185-11-2 $16.95

BLUE POPPY ESSAYS: 1988 Translations and Ruminations on Chinese Medicine by Flaws, Chace et al, ISBN 0-936185-10-4 $18.95

A HANDBOOK OF TRADITIONAL CHINESE DERMATOLOGY by Liang Jian-hui, trans. by Zhang Ting-liang & Bob Flaws, ISBN 0-936185-07-4 $14.95

A HANDBOOK OF TRADITIONAL CHINESE GYNECOLOGY by Zhejiang College of TCM, trans. by Zhang Ting-liang, ISBN 0-936185-06-6 (2nd edit.) $21.95

FREE & EASY: Traditional Chinese Gynecology for American Women 2nd Edition, by Bob Flaws, ISBN 0-936185-05-8 $15.95

PRINCE WEN HUI'S COOK: Chinese Dietary Therapy by Bob Flaws & Honora Lee Wolfe, ISBN 0-912111-05-4, $12.95 (Published by Paradigm Press, Brookline, MA)

TURTLE TAIL & OTHER TENDER MERCIES: Traditional Chinese Pediatrics by Bob Flaws ISBN 0-936185-00-7 $14.95

THE DAO OF INCREASING LONGEVITY AND CONSERVING ONE'S LIFE by Anna Lin & Bob Flaws, ISBN 0-936185-24-4 $16.95

FIRE IN THE VALLEY: The TCM Diagnosis and Treatment of Vaginal Diseases by Bob Flaws ISBN 0-936185-25-2 $16.95

HIGHLIGHTS OF ANCIENT ACUPUNCTURE PRESCRIPTIONS trans. by Honora Lee Wolfe & Rose Crescenz ISBN 0-936185-23-6 $14.95

ARISAL OF THE CLEAR: A Simple Guide to Healthy Eating According to Traditional Chinese Medicine by Bob Flaws, ISBN #-936185-27-9 $8.95

CERVICAL DYSPLASIA & PROSTATE CANCER: HPV, A HIDDEN LINK? by Bob Flaws, ISBN 0-936185-19-8 $23.95

PEDIATRIC BRONCHITIS: ITS CAUSE, DIAGNOSIS & TREATMENT ACCORDING TO TRADITIONAL CHINESE MEDICINE trans. by Gao Yu-li and Bob Flaws, ISBN 0-936185-26-0 $15.95